OUR ALTERED

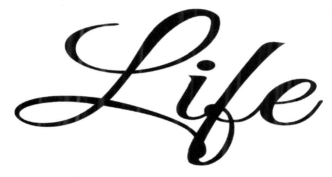

A MOTHER'S HEARTBREAK AND THE BOYS WHO SAVED HER

Charlene Beswick

To the lost mother I was and to those
who are still finding their way through
an unexpected but magical altered life.
Charlie x

Contents

Something is Wrong

"Your son has been born with half a face."

Okay, so that's not exactly what the consultant said, but it's basically what it boiled down to.

I had undergone an emergency caesarean a couple of hours earlier and had delivered twin boys. I had assumed that they were healthy. Why wouldn't they be? I don't smoke, hadn't drunk alcohol, ate well and never, not once, did I think I'd have anything other than two perfectly-formed, healthy children. But now I was being told otherwise.

Mark, my partner, was sitting to my left having just come back from making all the customary phone calls to announce the safe arrival of two boys. The midwife had popped her head into my cubicle while he had been gone and said that she'd come back when Mark was with me. I remember that her smile made me feel uneasy for a moment, but it passed as quickly as it came. I was still 'fuzzy' from the drugs and very tired, and so I dismissed my brief concern.

Once Mark was with me, the consultant came and sat at the foot of the bed, and Sarah, a lovely midwife about the same age as me, sat next to him, to my right. I remember being aware that she was watching me intently. Now I know why.

The consultant, Dr Mona, explained that twin one (Oliver) was fine, but twin two (Harry) had some problems. I can still see the way that Dr Mona drew an imaginary line down the centre of his face with his hand and swept it across to the left side as if he were erasing what was there. I processed it all in painfully slow motion, as if I were dreaming. His voice was muffled like he was talking to me underwater. I could hear the odd word, dulled by my delayed understanding and the pounding in my ears. At the same time, he was mentioning something about no eye, a small, under-developed ear, no nostril, a short and slanted jaw. He mentioned Golden something syndrome and hemi something or other. I now know these to be Goldenhar syndrome and Hemifacial Microsomia – different terms for similar conditions. Associated with this condition are heart defects, spinal problems and brain damage, but it was too early to know how severely Harry had been affected. He'd also been born with only one artery in his umbilical cord instead of two and the implications of this were, again, unknown at that time.

Dream. Bad dream. Thick, thick fog. What?

I remember looking from Dr Mona to Mark repeatedly as he told us the news like a person would look to a translator for help understanding a foreign language. I couldn't process this information. Not us. Not me. No. I felt as though I was drowning. This wasn't what was supposed to happen. Parents were told the weight of their babies. That it was time to hold and cuddle them. To gaze into their little eyes and pour themselves into their perfect creation feeling – an elation beyond anything they had ever known. It must be a mistake.

I sat perfectly still, frozen in that moment that I would relive for years to come. All I could whisper as fat, slow tears rolled down my face was, "I'm sorry. I'm sorry." No hysterical outbursts or sobbing convulsions. Just a paralysis of disbelief and guilt.

Despite being shocked and stunned, I found the guilt overwhelming. Mark squeezed my hand and told me I had nothing to be sorry for. Dr Mona also assured me that it wasn't due to anything that I had or hadn't done throughout the pregnancy, but I couldn't think anything else. When did it all go wrong?

Think, Charlene. Think. What did you do? What have you done to your child?

Hot on the tail of guilt came a much darker emotion. Fear. Dr Mona sat in front of me, describing a baby who only had half a face and, for all we knew, no quality of life ahead of him, and yet I was expected to love him. But what if I couldn't? What if I couldn't look at him, let alone hold him or bond with him? What if I was repulsed by this strange looking baby that I'd not expected or prepared for? Surely everyone would know just by looking at me. I wasn't the mother this boy needed.

When Sarah asked if I wanted to see him, I was absolutely terrified. Seeing him was the last thing that I wanted to do at that moment, but I said yes. What else could I say? What sort of cold, hard, unfeeling, wicked (feel free to add your own adjectives) person would I have been to admit my fears to anyone? It's only now when I reflect on those moments that I realise they were perfectly normal.

By now I had called the one person who I felt had the magical power to make this all right for me, to hold me through my nightmare and shush it all away. I don't remember what I said to my mum on my phone in the hospital bed. I know that I whispered, partly because only a thin curtain separated us from a ward full of mothers I no longer had anything in common with, partly because I knew that the alternative to whispering would drain me of any bit of energy I now had left. I think I said, "Something is wrong," and I cried. Mum left work immediately to come to us.

Many years later, when I faced all these feelings in the safe space of a therapeutic setting, I pictured a vase. Beautiful, big and colourful, but it had been smashed into hundreds of pieces. Every fragment had been retrieved and painstakingly reassembled so to all the world it still looked like the proud vase it once was. It still did the same job, but it was a fragile version of its former self. Changed forever. That moment, that day, was when my vase tipped off the edge of its table, hit the floor and shattered.

I don't know how long it was before the wheelchair came to take me to the Special Care Baby Unit (SCBU). The excitement that had filled me fewer than 24 hours ago felt like someone else's now, and all I had left was fear, dread and a sickness in the pit of my stomach. I forced a smile and got in the wheelchair. It was time to meet my boys.

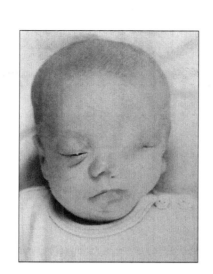

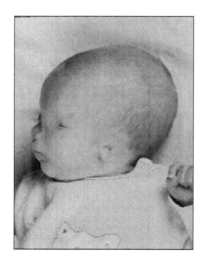

Introducing Charlene

Before I explain how the events following the birth of my boys affected me, I want to give you an idea of the person I was before I became a mum. It will make sense later – I'm not just being self-indulgent, I promise!

I've always been a chatterbox, an entertainer and an organiser. As a very young child, I used to sing on buses and encourage the other passengers to join in as if we were all going on holiday. I would run around aisles in the supermarket, returning to my mum and nan with price labels stuck all over my nose, only to hear them giggling at me. (There's nothing quite like thinking back to the days before bar codes and technology to make oneself feel old!) At my second cousin's birthday party, having played some games, I apparently rounded up all her guests, clapped my hands for attention and announced, "Right, let's open the presents now." I was five – a child full of mischief, humour and imagination who loved to make the people around me happy.

My parents had a difficult marriage, and when my father left my younger brother and me, I naturally adopted the role of looking after Mum. On one occasion,

I remember wrapping my little arms around her as she cried after yet another argument with my father. I vividly recall wanting the hurt to stop for her, to make it better somehow. I felt very protective of her even as a four-year-old, and as a result grew up quickly, choosing to be in adult company rather than with my peers if it meant that I was near her.

Don't get me wrong, I loved my childhood. I have wonderful memories of being adored and cherished by my mum, my nan and my grandad, and our bond was very strong, but striving to make the people around me happy is the legacy of my childhood. I worked hard at school, college, part-time and full-time jobs. This is not to say that I'm perfect, far from it, but anything I've done, I've given it 100% to ensure that I didn't let anyone down and made the people who matter proud of me.

This conviction applied to being a good mother, too, so when I gave birth to my twin boys two months early by emergency C-section only to discover that one of them had serious problems, it shook my foundations, my very understanding of who I was. How could I be the best partner and mother that I could be when I had failed *so* massively?

The impact of this will become apparent later, but I want to make it clear now that my future sadness and frustrations would be with me as much as 'fate' or 'science' or whatever other explanations were given to us. Ultimately, my search for the answers to "Why us?" would distract me from my most important mission – being a mum.

It took me almost two years to accept that something had been holding me back from loving my boys unconditionally and sharing a bond like the one I had with my own mum growing up. Me. And I've spent years putting that right and giving motherhood everything that my boys, and I, deserve.

When the boys were about 20 months old, I went to the hairdressers and read a magazine article about a woman whose son had been born with Treacher Collins syndrome. This meant that he had very little facial structure at all. She said something like, "When I held him, I just thought he needs me and I love him". She said that his problems weren't an issue for her at all, and I found myself wondering whether she was a very good liar, still in denial or superhuman? I couldn't empathise with her at all. In fact, my initial feelings were quite the opposite.

But far from making me feel like a terrible human being (let alone mother), her words made me realise that we're all different and that those differences aren't a bad thing. I'm glad that woman bonded with her son, but I thought about any new mums who would have read her story while struggling to come to terms with a baby who had been born with problems or complications. I wondered how the woman's story would have made them feel. I wondered because I knew how it would have made me feel in those early days. And those wonderings brought me to writing this book.

This is an account from the point of view of a mother who did struggle; for whom the bonding process and acceptance weren't instant and overwhelming. How much it would have meant to me to talk to somebody in the early weeks, who was prepared to be brutally honest and open. I think that would have helped me, and I hope that my story will help any struggling mother to realise that the darkness in the early weeks does pass and that it's not the end. Granted, the story for them, as it was for me, will be different to the one they imagined, but even tales with a twist can have a happy ending.

A Perfect Pregnancy

I had *loved* being pregnant! Apart from the fact that my once modest boobs resembled a couple of melons and my bladder shrank to the size of a grape (I never knew that just looking at liquid could have me dashing to the loo), I'd never felt better.

To say that we were shocked to discover that I was carrying twins is an understatement. I had been experiencing severe pain around my pelvis and so my GP referred me for a scan to rule out an ectopic pregnancy. I hoped and prayed that everything was OK. I was only seven weeks pregnant, this baby was barely more than a cluster of cells, and yet I already felt responsible for and protective of it. I can still remember lying on the couch in the Early Pregnancy Assessment Unit, the sonographer concentrating on the screen in front of her as she rolled the transducer wand over my jelly-covered belly.

"Have you been feeling sick at all?" she asked.

"No, not really." Smug tone – not even morning sickness, not me. "I feel fine, why?"

She turned the screen to me at that point. "Because you're carrying twins."

There was no denying two little sacs and two thumping heartbeats pounding away on the screen in front of us.

"*Now* I feel sick!" Panicked stare in Mum's direction. Then I burst into tears.

Once I was calm, I called Mark to tell him that everything was fine and that 'they' were waving.

Pause from his end.

"*They?*"

The panic and the shock, however, soon turned to excitement, and other than the worry of how we would afford double of everything, we couldn't wait to become a family. I remember Mark stroking my stomach one night before I got into the shower and smiling at the as yet bump-free home of our children, gently murmuring, "We're a team now." I felt blessed.

When I had a heavy bleed at 10 weeks, my mum drove me straight to the hospital. I sat still in the car for the journey and let tears roll down my face, laying my hands protectively across my stomach and silently begging, "Hang on, babies." To be told that everything looked fine and that I only needed to rest was an immense relief, and I think the scare made me appreciate my pregnancy even more.

As a passenger on a journey to Chester one Saturday with my mum and sister, I suddenly felt the strangest sensation in my stomach, like butterflies fluttering within me. I was only 14 weeks pregnant, but my babies were on the move and I was in awe of the miracle that was taking place inside my body. I treasured those moments, picturing my two babies wriggling together and enjoying the special time when I had them to myself, marvelling at the fact that two little people were camped out in my uterus for a while. I even sang to them in the bath, which may explain why they decided to arrive eight weeks early! John Denver's *Annie's Song* was my favourite, and one night the babies wriggled and kicked with the music. I felt our 'bond' grow through moments like that.

From early in the pregnancy I was convinced that I was carrying at least one boy. When the 20-week scan showed one dainty, clear side profile and one less defined profile, we hypothesised that we'd have a 'chunky monkey' boy and a delicate girl. Now, I know that the side profile of lumps and bumps was actually Harry's underdeveloped left side, but no one mentioned anything to us and so the excitement continued. Ignorance, most certainly, is bliss.

When I was around 25 weeks pregnant, I visited the Birmingham NEC Baby Show with my brother-in-law's girlfriend. It was a great day, full of inspirational ideas, creative solutions to everyday baby challenges that I hadn't even thought of yet and beaming faces. The excitement and anticipation was tangible as mothers paraded their bumps proudly and friends and partners chatted away.

We looked for the 4D scan stall for ages, but we inevitably got distracted by the other stalls and freebies. By the time we actually found it, the lady on the stall had just packed the machine away. I was incredibly disappointed – I wanted to see my babies' faces in the middle of the NEC with everyone looking on, pointing and cooing at the mum with the twins. I desperately wanted to catch a glimpse of the mini people who were living and breathing within me so that I could go home and tell everyone.

Now, looking back, I often wonder what would have happened if I *had* seen my babies' faces for the first time in the middle of the NEC. What if I had caught a glimpse of the mini people living and breathing within me? What would I have done, said or felt? I was disappointed for weeks because I had missed that opportunity, but I have felt grateful for years for the same reason.

See You on the Other Side

I felt so proud to be having twins. Blessed and privileged. Most people only managed one, but me? Oh, I was having *two*! My friends would laugh and say, "You don't do jobs by halves, do you?" I felt like Super Mum already. I did everything to make sure that my babies had the very best start, and other than feeling queasy in the evenings and craving salt and vinegar crisp butties and pint after pint of fresh, cold milk, I felt wonderful.

We imagined our life with the kids: strolling along and being stopped by strangers who would reach into their buggy and admire the two beaming little smiles. Having one of those informal action shot family photograph sessions. Baby groups with other mums and days out with other parents. Swapping stories of teething nightmares and sleep and weaning. Playing and laughing with our children. Sorting out the usual sibling squabbles, but observing with satisfaction the bond of friendship between our children which would stand the test of time, knowing that they would always have each other. Sharing stories of first dates. Counselling the traumas of first broken hearts. First holidays. Together.

Perfect. It felt amazing. Nothing more than any parent dreams of, expects and, now I realise, completely takes for granted.

I can honestly say that I never ever imagined or contemplated a life for me and my family that was anything other than 'normal'.

I joined the Twins and Multiple Births Association (TAMBA) and met many fantastic mums-to-be through online messages and emails. It was an excellent forum for tips and advice, and generally to let off steam to other multiple mums who were going through similar things.

Sometimes the topics diverged from baby talk and messages would be posted about relationship, intimate or embarrassing issues (none were mine, of course), and faceless online friends would come to the rescue with serious advice, sarcastic humour and lots of support. Reading and posting messages became a bit of an addiction, and when my waters broke, I made sure I logged on and posted a message ending with *see you on the other side*. I was only 32 weeks pregnant, but because we had found out that I was pregnant so early, it felt like we had waited forever. We didn't give any thought to the fact that the babies were premature; just that they were finally on their way to meet us.

The Boys' Birth

A friend of mine once told me about a conversation she'd heard at work. A pregnant colleague had said that she didn't mind if she had a boy or a girl just as long as it was healthy.

After the pregnant lady had left, my friend's boss had raised an eyebrow, tilted his head and asked, "And what if it's not healthy? What then?"

The assumption seems to be that you can love a healthy boy or girl, but what happens to that unconditional love when a baby is born with problems? It's an interesting point, and certainly not one that I had ever considered.

My waters broke at home on Wednesday 29 June 2005 at around 6.30pm following my regular 'granny nap'. Oh, how I loved those hours of guilt-free dribbling on the sofa!

The nurse at the hospital asked if I could have just urinated.

"Erm. No!"

I'd wet myself once when I was 15. Miles from home, laughing like a hyena with my best friend in a field, I had peed in my shell suit. This felt very different.

On inspection, the nurse assured me that nothing was happening but that I should stay in for a couple of weeks to get to 34 weeks gestation. However, by the early hours of Thursday my contractions were coming thick and fast. My cervix was examined regularly and I was making good progress towards delivering my boys naturally. That was until the hospital staff realised that Twin One was breach and I'd have to have an emergency C section almost immediately.

Becky, a fantastic midwife, handed me my phone at around 5am and told me to ring Mark and ask him to get to the hospital. Apparently I was too relaxed in my tone and so Becky took the phone off me to add some urgency to the situation, telling him to get there as soon as he could.

"No time to stop off for McDonald's breakfast!"

I hadn't wanted a caesarean. I had wanted the pain, the tears, the satisfaction of pushing my boys into the world and comparing stories of horror and triumph with other mothers afterwards. Hell, I even welcomed the perineum stiches and piles! I wanted Mark to witness me bringing our children into the world and love me in a way he had never felt before. But if it was best for the babies then I knew I had no choice.

One minute I was sucking on gas and air for dear life, and the next minute Katherine, the registrar, announced the arrival of my twins. Two boys. Oliver first at 6.33am. He loves to hear the actual words of announcement as he came into the world: "This one's got three legs! Happy birthday, Oliver." Followed by Twin Two three minutes later. Harry or George? We had struggled on this one, but settled on Harry.

Despite my midwife telling me not to panic if I didn't hear them cry instantly, I panicked anyway. As one of them whimpered followed by the next, I breathed a huge sigh of relief. Our boys were here.

Mark caught a quick glimpse of Oliver but told me that Harry was covered more by the blanket so he only saw a portion of his face. We weren't too worried by their rapid transfer to Special Care as they were premature, and we knew that they would be small: 3lb 9oz each. So within a few moments they were gone, leaving me to be sewn up and digest the amazing news with Mark. We were parents!

Thrilled, on the most incredible high, but thoroughly exhausted, I slept deeply back on the ward. Apparently, I snored, *loudly*. Classy! When I woke up, Mark had gone to make some phone calls and let everyone know the news.

It was 10.30am. When he came back, he sat to my left, and shortly afterwards we were joined by Dr Mona and Sarah.

Then Dr Mona delivered his news.

Unbearable Guilt

Seeing the boys for the first time is a bit of a blur. I was still trying to process what Dr Mona had told us. Part of me was terrified, the other part of me was numb. No part of me was happy or excited. That is never how you should feel as you meet your children for the first time. Ergo, added guilt.

Our boys were tiny, and covered in wires and tubes attached to machines that were bleeping and flashing numbers, giving information in a language we couldn't yet understand. These tiny scraps of people were so close to me yet so far away behind the equipment, the noises and my fear. I felt lost, and everything I did felt surreal. Like I was watching someone else do it instead. I was aware of what I *should* be feeling and I was acutely aware of how I wasn't feeling – like a 'mother'.

But, of all the emotions that I initially felt, the guilt was so intense and so unbelievably dark that words are completely inadequate to express it. What had I done to my boy? Everything ached. My throat ached from holding a golf ball sized lump of suppressed sobs; my head ached from the information I was trying to absorb; my body ached from an evening of no sleep and the surgery that followed; and my heart ached. It ached for the life I had dreamed of that was slipping through my fingers like grains of sand on a beach; for Mark whom I had failed; for my boy whom I had damaged; for my fractured self. All the while I was watching the mouths of nurses and doctors move and hearing nothing but mumbles.

I saw Harry twice before he was transferred to Hope Hospital in Salford to help with his breathing and for further investigations. Beyond being wheeled towards Special Care, I have little recollection now of our first meeting. I have little recollection of *anything* in the first few hours after the news had hit me like a bus.

The second time was in the early hours of Friday morning before he was transferred. He was in an incubator which could be lowered enough for me to see him from my wheelchair, and I waited with my heart pounding in my chest as the whirling machine brought him down to my level. He was lying on his stomach, facing away from me so I didn't see his face much at all, but for a brief moment he wrapped his tiny, perfectly formed hand around my finger. Time froze. I remember staring at the scene before me and thinking how incredibly beautiful that little hand was, and then he was gone. I was devoid of any reaction at all.

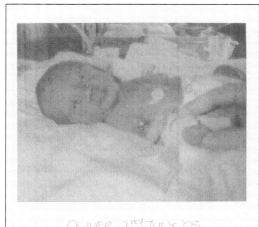

OLIVER 2nd JULY '05

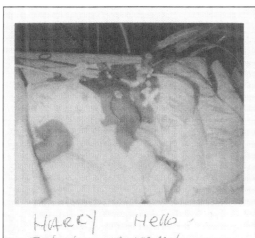

HARRY   Hello
30/6/05 MUMMY

Bonding with Oliver

I lay in my bed on the ward with Oliver next door in Special Care. Meanwhile, Harry was miles away in Salford where I stood no chance of getting to know him. And I wasn't exactly sure if or how I would ever do this. I lay and watched other mothers come back from the labour wards, cuddling their babies. In the night I lay, eyes open, listening to the gentle grunts and snuffles of the new-borns and the soft tones of their mothers comforting them. Proud mothers. Good mothers. Proper mothers. That was one of the hardest things for me in the first few days.

Something else that I wasn't prepared for, which sounds comical now, was the wind. I lay in bed, sore and tired, with gentle yet firm movements inside me, tricking me into thinking that I was still carrying my babies. Tormenting me. I wondered if all women felt this, or just me. Was this what loss felt like? A shadow of a memory replaying over and over where there was only emptiness – both physically and emotionally.

As the days ticked by, I got to know Oliver. I sat with him from the pre-dawn haze of another sleepless night until my eyes were too heavy and I had to leave his side. I watched over his tiny body and tried to imagine him and Harry being inside me. It was amazing to think that they had ever been there.

Initially, the oxygen mask which looked far too big for his tiny face, the tubes that seemed to come from everywhere and the monitors that constantly bleeped scared me and were a massive barrier between Oliver and me, but I soon got used to the sounds and the meanings of the alarms. I knew when to ignore them, when to wait for a member of staff to reset them and when to worry. I was even beginning to understand and use the technical terms.

As it all became familiar, everything felt calmer and safer somehow. I rationalised that the equipment was only doing what my own body would have done had the boys not been born so early. I trusted the machines and the staff to nourish and protect the boys better than I trusted myself anymore. I also knew that whatever was happening for Oliver in Macclesfield was also happening in the SCBU in Salford for Harry.

Around day four, the SCBU staff at Macclesfield rang Hope Hospital and I spoke to the nurse caring for Harry. I was able to understand all of the technical terms that she used to explain how he was doing, and I followed the conversation with a detached acceptance and understanding as she told me about his progress.

At the end of the conversation, she said, "Don't worry. We're giving him lots of cuddles. He's a very cuddly boy."

I broke down. As I nodded silently, unable to thank her, one of the staff took the phone from me and I dissolved into tears in the arms of another nurse. I was so grateful that Harry was being cuddled and loved, but the thought that someone else was giving this affection to him when it should have been me, that someone already knew my boy while he was still a stranger to me, left me with a physical pain.

Why Us? Why Harry?

It felt wonderful and awful at the same time to be bonding with Oliver. I was only too aware that every cuddle, touch, loving gaze and smell of his innocent, vulnerable, tiny, perfect body in my arms were crucial times for us that Harry was missing. I wondered and worried if I would be able to love Harry like I did his brother when he was transferred back. Did I even want that day to happen? More guilt.

I pushed myself as hard as possible to get mobile. It was frustrating to have my mind, thoughts and energy hampered by a sluggish go-slow body that was aching and sore, but on Sunday 3 July, Mark was allowed to take me to Hope Hospital to visit Harry.

Hope SCBU was vast with incubators everywhere. I remember thinking it looked like a scene from a science fiction film. It was darker and less peaceful than Macclesfield due to the number of staff popping in and out. It felt strange, but the bleeping monitors were familiar and reassuring.

Harry was lying on his stomach facing away from us when we arrived. He looked just like Oliver. Mark and my mum had been the first to see Harry, and I remembered her saying to me that he had a broad back and strong shoulders. I saw that she was right.

A geneticist met us at the side of the incubator and asked a lot of questions. Did we have any history of birth defects in either of our families? Were Mark and I related at all? I was confused as Dr Mona had told me that Goldenhar wasn't a genetic syndrome, but I answered the questions in a numb, distant fog as I sat and stared at the stranger who was my boy, wondering again how I had managed to cause all of this.

I was so terribly afraid to hold him that the fear gripped me from within. He was tiny and frail and unfamiliar, and I was unsure how I would cope looking at him when all I would see was my failure. I'd love to tell you every thought and every emotion I felt during that first visit, but if I'm honest, and that is my intention, it's all a bit of a blur now. I know that I cried as I watched him lie in that incubator with the UV light on him for his jaundice, and I cried as his floppy body was scooped out of the incubator and placed in my arms.

My heart was pounding as I was finally faced with the reality of the doctors' descriptions and my own imagination. My boy looked back at me and I took short glances to take in the absence of his face. I don't recall acknowledging to myself that his perfectly formed side was actually very pretty, which is a shame as it really is beautiful. Mark took my photograph as I held our son for the first time and I smiled, but inside I was broken. Part of me wanted to scream; part of me had retreated to some quiet, still darkness and wanted to stay there forever.

I'm sure that I felt happy at times. I must have done, but those first few weeks were saturated with grief for the future that we felt we'd been robbed of and for the fulfilling, rewarding and precious elation after the birth that I had imagined, but never experienced. Instead, sadness overwhelmed me.

In the car on the way back to Macclesfield Hospital, I was aware that I was crying, but I could also hear a shrill, relentless shrieking coming from somewhere outside of me. It took me a while to connect the two. I screamed through my tears and could barely catch my breath.

Mark drove and I just howled beside him. God knows what he must have been feeling. He had been visiting Harry in Manchester and Oliver and me in Macclesfield every day. He must have been exhausted, and now he was listening to his fiancée wail next to him, sharing his fears but alone at the same time.

I remember wanting to say that Harry had beautiful eyes, but I could only say eye. I wanted to say that I didn't see his differences because he was my boy and I loved him so they didn't matter, but in the early days, his differences were all that I could see. They did matter. They really did.

I asked Mark, "Why us?" and "Why Harry?" He had just as many questions as I did and no one had any answers. I thought about my pregnancy so hard that my head ached. I must have eaten something, or pushed myself too hard. Maybe it happened when I bled.

Friends and family would tell me that it wasn't my fault, but it was like their voices were muffled and distant. I wanted to scream, "SHUT UP!" at them all as a rage like I'd never experienced before simmered and churned away among the fury of injustice and the hormones. At least if I were responsible, we'd have a reason. Blaming myself was surely easier than having no explanation. We wanted concrete answers from which we could move forward, but there were none for us to find.

At times, the darkness and the sorrow would wash over me like a tidal wave, so oppressive and heavy that it was physically hard to breathe and impossible to think anything other than, *what have I done to him?* On one occasion, I remember being in the car with Mark, calmly thinking, *if I died then all this would stop.* The only thing I could hear was static hissing. I hated myself so intensely. I expected Mark to hate me too, and convinced myself that some part of him actually did.

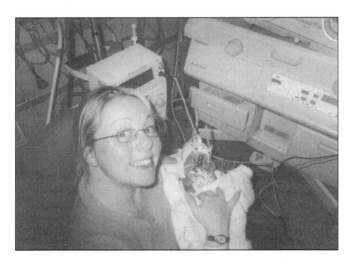

The Healing Words of an Expert

Back at Macclesfield, the staff were amazing. Rachel, the midwife who had been with me during the contractions only four nights and one lifetime ago, came into my cubicle one night and sat on the end of my bed. She'd had a few days off and had come to see how I was. She had rung the ward the day after the boys had been born to see how they were doing and said that she'd been in a vile mood all weekend, thinking about the injustice of it all.

Everyone else was trying hard to look on the positive side, to smile and avoid the subject of how unfair and crappy the whole situation was. Not feeling that I could vent my frustration meant that it festered inside me and tortured my quiet moments. So it was a miserable and wonderfully refreshing conversation that I had with Becky that Monday night, cross-legged by the light of my bedside lamp like girls on a sleepover.

Another nurse smiled politely as she filled my water jug one afternoon before telling me about her young nephew who had a false eye that he looked after well and with pride. It was nice to hear these tales, but as my auntie used to say, "There's no pain in the arse like *my* pain in the arse." And so, the nurse's kind, well-meaning tale, meant to offer hope for my boy's future, fell on the deaf ears of a lost and weary woman who was still absorbed in self-pity and panic. An absent eye, ear and nostril were going to be the tip of the iceberg for a baby who had done nothing to this cruel world but be born into it.

During my second visit to Hope Hospital I had a telephone conversation with Dave Kent, an ENT consultant who melted the ice that I was forming around myself in a way that no one else had been able to do. He called Harry my 'beautiful son', and I vividly remember what he said in his soothing yet assertive tone.

"I can promise you three things. First, if there is anything you want to know, you can call me. If I don't know the answers then I'll find someone who does. Secondly, we'll make sure that we have the best people in the country working with Harry. And thirdly," he paused here to make sure I was listening, "it wasn't your fault."

I remember him saying that it wasn't because of anything I had or had not done, and that he knew how much mothers blamed themselves. He assured me that I shouldn't.

I nodded silently on the end of the phone and whispered, "Thank you," as I cried. Even now, years later, my eyes still fill as I remember the words of an expert, not just a comforting friend or relative who was saying what I wanted to hear. It helped me immensely to drag myself through the vast and oppressive darkness of those first few weeks, and I shall always be grateful to Mr Kent.

*****

Introducing Oliver
and Harry

On the Tuesday after the boys had been born, I was allowed to go home. Just me. No babies, but lots of gifts, flowers and balloons, a sore belly full of wind and an ache inside. I had been reluctant to leave Oliver in hospital, despite trusting the expert care and attention that he would receive. But I missed Mark and I knew that both of us could be stronger together than either of us could be apart. On a more practical level, I was looking forward to a shower in my own bathroom and a good night's sleep in my own bed in the hope that I'd feel half human again.

I had watched so many women come and leave the ward with their babies. Off home to start the lives that I had been dreaming of with my children. I was happy for every single one of them, but with every pursed-lipped half smile that they cast in my direction as they said goodbye, I felt a twisting stabbing cramp in the pit of my stomach. Why did they get a healthy baby and I didn't? How dare they feel sorry for me? I'd got more than enough self-pity and I didn't need any more.

But they were well-meaning parting glances, and if I had been taking a healthy bundle of joy home and leaving a mum looking lost and lonely without her babies, I would have felt sorry for her too. And then I would have thanked my lucky stars that it had happened to her and not me. But that's human nature. We all want the simple life, and I'm no different.

What took me a long time to realise is that, in his own way, Harry is perfect. Perfectly sweet and kind and accepting of all those people who look normal to the rest of the world but who are cruel, judgemental and rotten inside. Give me a perfect soul any day.

Once I was home, one of the first things that I did was to log on to TAMBA. I had had dozens of messages of support and excitement to begin with, then some asking where I was a few days later. As I read my initial message it all felt like a very long time ago.

I took a deep breath and posted a new message: *Introducing Oliver and Harry... there's a 'but', though.* I poured my heart out to the friends I'd made who were waiting for my news. I explained as much as I knew and I remember crying as I typed that I loved my boy with all my sad heart. I didn't know if that was really true, or if I'd ever feel the joy and pride that other mums were writing about. I suddenly felt very isolated from the other members. I had nothing in common with them anymore.

Looking back, I think one of the most overlooked tragedies of the whole experience was that the shock and sadness and disappointment of Harry's problems meant that I never fully acknowledged or appreciated that I had had another son who was absolutely fine. I had Oliver in common with every other mother who'd had the child they expected. I just couldn't see it at the time. During moments when I sat cuddling Oliver in hospital, I would pour myself into his eyes and stroke every perfectly formed inch of his tiny body, but too often I would be thinking, *this is what Harry should be like* instead of feeling the elation of my beautiful, healthy boy. It was like Oliver's lack of problems was insignificant against the potential catalogue of issues facing Harry.

So I sat at my computer, feeling alone and appalled at myself for my incompetence at being unable to carry two healthy babies. Based on my performance as a mother so far, I doubted my ability to be a half-decent parent and I wondered how on earth I would get through the next day, let alone the future.

A Glimmer of Happiness

I remember the first day that Mark and I actually felt genuine happiness after the boys had been born. It was the day that Hope Hospital confirmed that Harry's kidneys, spine and heart had not been affected by the syndrome. Before then, people had tried to comfort us by saying that Harry had come to us because we were 'special parents'. We didn't want to be 'special parents' and I would spit the words out like poisonous venom. If I were to compile a Top 10 list of things *not* to say to parents like us, 'special' would definitely be in the top three. We wanted to be normal parents with two perfectly healthy babies like everybody else in the whole wide world. The self-pity made us exaggerate our own problems and forget the millions of other families in the same boat.

We didn't feel special or blessed, but that day we became aware that things could have been far worse for us and for Harry. We drove home, chatting as the car snaked through the hedge-flanked, winding roads about how our future would have looked if Harry had had those internal problems. I remember looking at Mark and smiling – *really* smiling. Not the superficial one I had perfected over the last week or so, but the kind that spreads up to your eyes and makes them shine.

And, taking a deep breath as if I had just surfaced from underwater, I said, "I actually feel happy."

He smiled back, squeezed my hand and agreed. It was the first time in what felt like an eternity that I had felt positive. Small steps. That's all we could take. And sometimes we took one step forwards and two steps back, but smiling was good. Smiling meant progress.

Bonding with Harry

The day Harry joined Oliver at Macclesfield was another good day for us. Apart from feeling relieved that the physical and emotional drain of travelling between the two hospitals was over, I felt excited to have my boys together. I was looking forward to seeing Harry, too. Until now it had only been Mark, Mum, me and the hospital staff who had seen him. Now, we would be introducing him to family and friends. I wondered what they would think of him and how I would cope.

Some visitors were more vocal about their feelings than others. I vividly remember one visitor saying, "Oh, Charlene! He's nowhere near as bad as you made out. I was expecting to see a monster, but he's not."

I wanted to shout, "Yes, yes! Monster, monster, monster! I get it," but I just bit my bottom lip and stared through welled up eyes into the incubator of Harry's neighbour, another premature baby who was patiently waiting for his visitors to arrive. Initially, I felt incredibly angry that someone should describe Harry as a monster, but this rage soon turned inward as I questioned the ways I had portrayed him. Had the language I'd used to describe him actually suggested that I saw Harry in that way?

In fact, I had never seen Harry like that. The only monster I saw in the whole situation was me. For failing to give Harry the life that Oliver would take for granted and for being unable to love them both equally and unconditionally. I thought about the words that we used to describe Harry's appearance and concluded that it wasn't what we'd said, but how the listener had interpreted it and built up a picture in their own mind. Looking back, I am pleased that people expected to see worse. They had a mental preparation time that I had never had.

Undoubtedly, Harry is much more than 'no eye, no eye socket, no ear or nostril and a short jaw' so I guess the description didn't do him justice. Now when I describe the syndrome, I add, "It sounds much worse that it looks. He's a real cutie", and when people agree and comment on how lovely he is, I trust that they're not just taking pity on us.

Having Harry at Macclesfield gave me a real chance to study him. The right hand side of his face was perfect in every way and very similar to Oliver's. However, the left hand side looked as if it had been rubbed out. To the top left of the bridge of his nose there was a bump of squishy tissue which lay diagonally across to where his eyebrow would have been. Below this was a smooth hollow space instead of an eye. He had the slit of an eye, but it was closer to his temple than to his nose. There were no surrounding eyelids, but a few lashes were clumped together in the far corner. The doctors wondered if there were remnants of the early stages of a developing eyeball beneath the surface, but warned us that if there was anything there, it would probably resemble a shrivelled pea and require early surgery to remove it.

His 'ear' was a tiny lobe, and although it was roughly in the right place, it looked just like a blob of skin. From the tip of Harry's nose out to the left looked like it had collapsed, and instead of a full nostril there was a tiny hole on a curved and featureless blank canvas.

The more I saw of Harry and cuddled him, the more familiar he and his differences became. The tight knot inside me loosened and I began to relax more. At Hope Hospital and initially at Macclesfield, I had felt quite strange whenever I forced myself to scrutinise both the perfection and the absence of his tiny face. I don't think that I ever felt repulsed, although I would totally understand if mothers in my situation did, but certainly there was a discomfort. I would have a searing pain as if part of me was physically retracting and tensing. It felt like the brief but precise pain of pulling a plaster off quickly. But after that sting came a dull ache and throb, followed by some small attempt to heal.

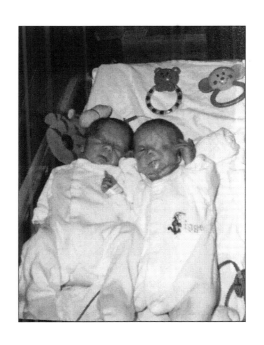

Daisy the Cow

The day after the boys had been born, I started expressing my milk. They were obviously too small and delicate to feed from me themselves, and so I saw this as me doing my best for them. While I was in hospital, I used the prehistoric looking electrical breast pump there – the assembly of which was so complicated that I felt like I was in training to rebuild a car engine. But it did the job.

As with everything I've ever done, I threw myself into providing the boys with the nourishment they needed. I expressed as much as I could every three to four hours. I didn't realise at the time that the more you express, the more you produce, so it didn't take long before my boobs had swollen to fill my armpits and ached to be relieved. Yet I persevered.

I even expressed through the night for the first couple of months. Mark would be snoring upstairs, and I would sit in the lounge in the dark while my electrical breast pump sucked and released my nipple in a poor imitation of the babies that my breasts had expected. No place was safe from the rhythmical groaning of my pump – Mark's parents' house; the hospital; lay-bys. 'Daisy the

Cow' became my new nickname. Humour is a powerful and comforting ally at times.

The nurses at the hospital had suggested that I look at a picture of the boys while I expressed to stimulate my hormones, but that felt too strange – a bit deviant to be releasing my energy while pouring myself into their images. If anything, thinking about them made expressing harder.

At home, I would flick through the television channels to amuse myself, but would often end up watching programmes about multiple births and babies. The same programmes that I had religiously watched in the name of research since we'd found out we were expecting twins. Now, I forced myself to watch them as some form of torture. I would stare at the screen as mothers went into labour and progressed, as I had done, only to be greeted by a couple of symmetrical crumpled little faces. Their lives were complete and their futures bright. Ours were scary and uncertain.

Sometimes I would feel positively furious with the lucky parents who were surely no better than us. Other times I would sit silently and sob. The ache and the grief of losing all my hopes and dreams would be so real that I wanted to curl up and let the world pass me by. Let someone else deal with my premature twins, my disfigured child. Just leave me alone.

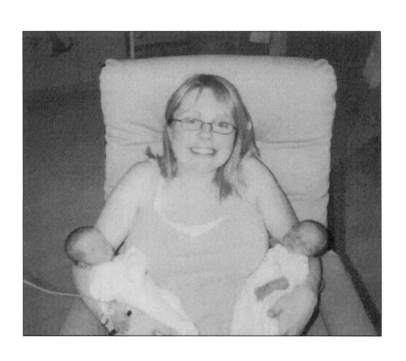

An Emotional Rollercoaster

Mum came to drive me to the hospital one morning during one of my sobbing episodes. As she came in, I remember literally falling into her arms. If ever a turn of phrase was appropriate, 'heartbreak' did it for me. My heart and my dreams were shattered and I had no idea how to begin to put it right. I resented the energy required to think about what Harry's and our future held when all other new mums were happily investing their time and energy into their new 'bundles of joy'. I was so very bitter. And jealous. I remember sobbing on the floor until I couldn't catch my breath, and Mum sat with her arms around me, as I had done for her as a small child.

It took a while for me to realise that I shouldn't fight these moments, but embrace them for what they were. My release. I had to allow myself time to cry and feel sorry for myself, but then I had to pick myself up, dust myself off and make it through the day. Just one at a time.

At the same time as battling my own feelings, thoughts and emotions, including the dreaded hormones that meant that previously 'soppy and ridiculous' TV adverts now had me sobbing into my Kleenex, I was conscious of the feelings of Harry's visitors. I remember my nan's first visit. My nan was my hero in life – the strongest, bravest and most incredible woman I have ever known.

I had worried about telling her that I was expecting twins, but when I did, she laughed and said, "Ooooooh, you little devil!" Her approval meant absolutely everything to me, so I was beyond terrified to introduce her to my Harry.

As she peered into the cots and marvelled at the tiny, vulnerable babies beneath the wires who had yet to grow into their baggy suits of skin, she was clearly wrestling with her natural instinct to cuddle and protect them. I stared intently at her eyes for any sign that my son and I were a disappointment to her. If she felt anything near disappointment, her gaze never betrayed it. I could see that she had the love and acceptance that I chased and found to be so elusive.

*****

Every day for four weeks, somebody would come to take me to the hospital. This meant having conversations with my chauffeurs about the boys and about how we were coping. I avoided the subject of the future, partly because it scared me and partly because we didn't know anything anyway. It was easier to be strong for other people when they got overwhelmed and upset about the unfairness of it all.

When visitors said that Harry's problems didn't matter and that he was still cute, I either smiled and tried to forget the comment or felt like punching them and screaming, "Don't pity us or talk such shit! Do you think the world is ready for this? This is *not* cute." In the first couple of weeks I really struggled to see Harry as a person behind the syndrome. I am not proud of the things I felt or thought, but I never hated him. I hated the world, the universe, God, myself, but I never hated Harry. I couldn't. I barely knew him. As I did get to know him and his little ways, the toxic feelings I had were slowly replaced by acceptance and love.

Each day our visitors would leave and I would sit in between the boys' plastic hospital cots, assisting with then actually doing and recording their feeds and changes. Mark would leave work and come to see his new family every day, and take me home without them.

It's amazing to think now how excited we used to get about their feeds. I would call Mark from outside and say, "He's had 10ml!" and he would be as thrilled as a parent who has just been told their toddler has taken their first steps. Now, the boys think nothing of gulping 10ml of medicine mid-run before dashing past me. But back then, 10ml through a gravity feed down a tube into their noses and then stomachs was a big deal.

Each day we visited them, something new had happened. Often we would find a Polaroid picture of them sharing a cot and looking up at the camera for us. The staff in the SCBU were truly amazing. Their support, understanding and skill, not just with babies or apparatus, but with families, are grossly under-recognised, but were immensely appreciated by us.

One day, we arrived to be greeted by unusually serious faces. The results of Harry's CT and MRI scans were back and Dr Mona wanted to discuss them with us. I was so very afraid.

We stood in the same tiny room that I'd met Harry in before his transfer to Hope. The room in which he'd wrapped his tiny hand around my strong, healthy finger as his introduction. That felt like a long time ago as we stood waiting for today's news.

I concentrated hard as Dr Mona flicked the light box on and placed Harry's scans on it. My eyes were hungry for every detail and ate each picture up, while my brain made a conscious effort to hear, understand and store every morsel of information that accompanied them.

The scans were amazing. We could see all of Harry's teeth as if he were a fully toothed toddler, and we stared at the images of his skull with curiosity and wonder. Whereas his right eye socket was a perfect hole in a mass of surrounding bone, the left socket was no more than a tiny gap. When I explain it to other people, I use the analogy of a cave in which the material surrounding the entrance has collapsed because there is nothing for it to form around. The absence of a half-hearted attempt at an eye was a relief because this meant that he wouldn't require early surgery.

What was interesting was the fact that there appeared to be a portion of an optic nerve to his missing eye. This was bittersweet news. To think that Harry had been so close to being spared the ordeal of years of hospital visits and procedures to achieve what nature would have accomplished in a matter of days felt cruel. Immediately we were asking about the possibility of popping a false eye in, plugging in the optic nerve, *et voila*! Vision. But Dr Mona was clearly no wiser than us.

In time, we would become the experts on Harry and the implications of his syndrome rather than the catalogue of professionals who had little experience of the various forms in which Goldenhar presents itself. But at that time, we were travelling in uncharted territory and had to be cautious not to make too many assumptions.

The scan showed no obvious damage to the formation of Harry's brain and confirmed that the lump of fatty tissue protruding from his forehead was just cartilage, not brain tissue trying to escape through a crack in his skull. We felt so relieved. No brain damage was great news. While I knew that the scan only told us about the brain's structure and not its function, it gave us hope, and really, that's all any of us have got.

I remember that I became very overwhelmed and emotional, and at some point in the conversation I lost sight of Harry's scans behind a mist of tears. I can't recall if I actually hugged Dr Mona, but I certainly wanted to.

When I came out of the room, my instinct was to go straight to Harry, who had become a little bit grizzly, and pick him up. I held him to me lengthways up the front of my chest as I tried to contain myself and calm my inner tremble. All of a sudden, he pushed himself away from my body, and for the first time in his life he stilled and stared right into me as if to say, "See, I will be fine. Don't be upset".

Moments like that were overwhelmingly beautiful and intense.

Bonding as a Family

It's difficult to describe the bond that I developed with my boys. Some days I would feel close to both of them and that I knew them. Other days, particularly on the days when the guilt prevented me from even looking at Harry, I would feel closer to Oliver. However, there were days when I felt like nothing more than a babysitter who happened to be spending time with premature twins called Oliver and Harry.

One day, Mark and I were sitting with the boys, and I vividly remember feeling myself emotionally withdraw and detach from the family as if having some sort of out of body experience, looking at the cheery father and troubled mother as they held an infant each. Mark saw a change in me and commented on it later. I couldn't explain it. I felt like they were somebody else's children and partner and I was just a spectator of their bonding. It did pass, but the feeling was intense and the aftermath left me feeling exhausted.

While the boys were still in Special Care, Mum told me about a woman who visited an elderly patient in the hospital where she worked. She said that this woman's young son had been born with a rare syndrome, lots of problems and had already had surgery. She would be a good person for Mark and me to talk to, so when we got a call one afternoon to say that she was on the ward, Mum suggested that we go up there to meet her.

Now you may think I'd have felt relieved to be on the way to meet a parent who had been where I was, but I didn't. I was nervous, and part of me didn't want to hear the stories of what lay ahead for us – despite my curiosity. Sometimes it's much easier to bury your head in the sand until you're made to face the reality of a life that's different.

Her son was lovely, running around the ward like any other toddler. I thought nothing of it until his mum said, "We were told he'd never walk, but look at him." I couldn't imagine helpless little Harry being a tearaway toddler, but I hoped that he would be. The mum told me all about her son's condition, his operations and the future as much as she knew at that point. It turned out that he also had Goldenhar syndrome, but had been affected in different areas. She talked in convoluted medical and technical terms that confused and frightened me. It was like listening to a foreign language. We're now fluent in cranio-facial jargon, but at that time it felt like another huge obstacle to overcome.

She warned me that the doctors would try to take over and said that it was important that we did what we felt was right for Harry. I wondered how on earth I would ever know what was right for him. I remember being amazed at how much spirit and strength she had and I questioned whether I was up to the challenges faced by a special needs mum.

*****

Back in Special Care, the boys were making good progress. They were feeding well and putting weight on and developing their own little personalities. Oliver was impatient and wanted a lot of attention, whereas Harry was more placid and enjoyed cuddles. I visited every day, as did Mark, and we formed some lovely relationships with the staff who felt as close as extended family.

Sometimes, as the boys got stronger and were gradually taken off their various monitors, I would sit in the family room with them both and we would cuddle and chat and watch television. I enjoyed those moments, knowing that they were practice sessions for me to be alone with the boys in preparation for their discharge. The thought filled me with excitement, and fear. In hospital, the staff were always on hand, day or night, to answer any questions or to give me advice or support. It was reassuring and safe in the SCBU, but as the boys improved, I knew we were taking up places needed by other poorly babies and frightened parents. I would see new arrivals and watch like a seasoned veteran as the parents and families jumped at the beeps and alarms of the monitors and were trained in the ways of handling their own baby.

Oliver was ready to come home slightly before Harry, but the staff at Macclesfield Hospital decided to keep the boys together until Harry was also strong enough. It didn't take long, and on Sunday 6 August we went to Macclesfield SCBC for the last time.

Coming Home

It was quite emotional to leave. Exciting and daunting. I hugged the staff as we put our tiny babies in their car seats. Harry weighted 4lb 9oz and Oliver weighted 5lb 1oz. Then we left. Nearly six weeks after my boys had been born, I finally achieved what I'd watched so many other families do – I took my babies home.

Back at home we existed in a parallel universe where days lasted for an eternity and comprised of feeding, sleeping and a wide variety of poo types (the boys', not ours). While I had been pregnant I had watched many top tips for parents of twins who were mastering the art of synchronised feeding. I did try to feed the boys at the same time, propped up on pillows as the programmes had demonstrated, but Harry required one-to-one attention and I don't even think I made it through one feed.

As it was, the boys took their feeds at staggered times anyway. Every three hours a hungry baby requested to be fed immediately. An hour and a half later, the other one would do the same. And repeat. All through the day. All through the night. It was tiring while I had Mark with me for the first two weeks, but being on my own took the exhaustion to a new level.

While Oliver was the baby most likely to projectile vomit across the room, Harry struggled to suck due to only having the one nostril. On a good day he would suckle away like a baby lamb on my expressed milk and finish the bottle within half an hour. However, if he had so much as the snuffles, he would search frantically for the teat, take two sucks and then push it away, gasping for his breath. One feed could take up to an hour and a half, and he would finish just in time for Oliver to start again. Thankfully I had my mum and nan close by to supply another pair of hands to feed, change, nurse and generally entertain whichever twin wasn't with me.

There would be mornings when, having watched the sun rise yet again, I would lie perched on the very edge of the sofa, my cold and aching back facing the window and the two boys snuggled on the sofa in front of me. I would hear the back door unlock and light footsteps creep across the laminate flooring towards the lounge. My angel, my nan would pop her head over me and the bundle of arms and legs. She would either take my place on the edge of the sofa or gently take one of the wide awake and restless boys. Most mornings I looked like I had been on a 48-hour drinking binge and was fighting to keep my eyes open.

Even when Harry did sleep, it didn't mean that Mark and I did. In the evenings, Oliver's Moses basket was positioned at the foot of our bed and Harry's was to the right. Against usual recommendations, Harry had to sleep on his front, and we had to elevate the mattress slightly as he was prone to bringing his milk back up, often down his nose. We had been reassured by the doctors at the hospital that his palate was intact, but professionals who visited once we were home often questioned this and so we were unsure. We were aware that even common actions for a baby like Harry, such as being sick down his nose, could have sinister implications. We checked on him every 20 minutes through the night, taking it in turns to have blocks of a few hours' sleep. I was aware that Mark was working through the days and tried to do as much as possible without him, but I think even Superwoman would have struggled to juggle a full-time bedside vigil and two hungry babies.

Macclesfield Hospital provided us with an apnoea alarm, which was attached to Harry's stomach. It would go off if it detected that he had stopped breathing – I think the intention was to provide us with some peace of mind and give him some extra protection. As much as I hoped it would never go off, I was prepared to jump out of bed with the reflexes of a ninja in the event that it did. Thankfully it never actually went off, although I'm sure I imagined hearing it more than once. It was a bit like someone saying, "There's a bomb under your car, but just drive normally until it explodes." Relaxing was never going to happen.

As tiring and relentless as the daytime feeds felt, it was the night time feeds that I struggled with the most. Those 3am feeds when the floor upstairs vibrated with the rumbles of Mark's contented snores and I sat shivering on the sofa. Nervous of heating bottles of expressed milk in the microwave, I would boil the kettle, fill a jug with boiling water and pop the bottle in for a few moments. Those few moments were all I needed to put the jug on the wooden floor in the lounge and kick it over, scalding one foot and hopping madly on the other while swearing profusely. If I had a pound for every time I did that, I would be rich!

Once mastitis had ravaged my breasts and the boys were on formula milk, I was happier to warm it in the microwave, and that is the tale of how my poor, weary boobs and tortured toes survived.

The Good, the Bad and the Downright Stupid

About a week after we brought the boys home I had my first visit from the health visitor. I was tired, grumpy, emotional and, quite frankly, still trying to get my head around all that was happening. Her infantile tone and pity head tilt meant that our initial introduction didn't start well.

She knew my son had 'Golden something' but she had never heard of it before and asked me to explain what it was. I told her what I knew, despite not understanding it fully myself.

She then followed this up with, "Do you think it was something that you did?"

How I restrained myself from hitting her I will never know. Instead I asked her to leave, and had rung the surgery to insist she was never sent to my house again before she had even left my drive. I was furious, and at the same time terrified that this wasn't going to be the only time I would be faced with that question. Self-pity was a force to be reckoned with at times and I did struggle, but I had to try and focus on the bigger picture. Not the future, just the normal things that needed doing in that day.

Some days, though, I couldn't manage it. I would collapse beneath the sheer weight of "Why me?" and "Why us?" On one occasion, my mum's partner at the time told me to snap out of it and be positive. My acerbic reply almost cut the head off his shoulders. I knew that I should be feeling positive. I understood that days like this couldn't last forever, but I reserved the right to have the odd day when I ignored all the things I *should* do and did what I needed to do: have a good cry.

One morning, after a particularly bad night, I lay on the sofa staring at Harry in the large travel cot in the brightest corner of the bay window, content with his toys. There were so many extra things that we had to do for Harry: extra attention through the night; physiotherapy exercises to encourage him to use the muscles in the left side of his neck so that they didn't waste away. Everything took longer and required more conscious effort, and there were some days when I was just tired of it. I knew it was important, but I resented the effort that it required when I wanted to be investing that effort into the other needs the boys had.

Mum came in to give me a kiss and I remember whispering, "I feel like I have half a baby," and crying in a numb calmness – ashamed to be even thinking it, let alone saying it. As always, she held me through those moments, and as always, it passed as quickly as it came and I brushed the sadness off.

The second health visitor who came to see me was fantastic. She had done her homework on Harry's syndrome and came with the positive 'can do' attitude that I needed. Never once did I feel that she judged me, despite the fact that on more than one occasion I opened the door (before the curtains) to her at 10am still wearing my pyjamas. If ever I did talk about my worries – Harry's awful sleep pattern; his recurring ear infections during which I was helpless to comfort him; the lack of time to myself to get even basic things done – she always listened and came back with a solution.

She referred us to the disability sleep team who came to offer advice on Harry's bedtime routine; she spoke to his paediatrician and arranged for Harry to have grommets fitted to his one ear; and she arranged for a perfect stranger to come to my house once a week to give me time to myself.

Now this last point was a big issue for me. Someone I didn't know would look after my boys with their khaki green nostril-rotting nappies, projectile vomiting and complex needs, and I would be leaving her to it for an hour? I wasn't sure.

Then I met Annette.

We spent an hour at our house with my boys and permanent sidekick – Nan. I wondered what Annette would think of Harry, but she seemed to see only the little boy and not the syndrome. In no time at all she felt like part of the family. I looked forward to her Thursday visits, and for over six months, that hour was my sanity – time to relive the granny nap with synchronised snoring and dribbling in bed; time to nip into town for nothing in particular and manage to spend money on half a dozen items I didn't need (although that's a genetic curse passed on from my mother); time to wrap

Christmas presents upstairs that I could hide well and find again in February (see previous curse). Soon, I wondered how I'd ever managed without her, and why I had worried.

As I look back on our journey, it seems that many of the decisions I felt the most apprehensive about turned out to be the best ones I made.

*****

Just as I had with Annette, I often feared what people would think when they saw Harry. By now, I was becoming familiar with the absence on his left side of all that was perfect on his right. Over time, I trained my eyes to focus on his right hand side, not because I couldn't bear to look at his left side, but because there really was no point. Any expressions or reactions were shown on the right side of his face.

It wasn't until I lifted him to the mirror when he was older to show him his reflection and my eye was drawn across to the side where there was only skin and bumps that I realised I had trained myself like this. It had never been a conscious decision. At times I marvel at how amazing a human brain can be in protecting the fragile mind of its owner.

I took photographs of the boys all the time – as they played; as I cuddled them; as they rocked back and forth in their motorised swings, sometimes falling asleep and flopping over. Capturing action shots of Oliver was easy. It was simple to get him to look towards the camera, and as the boys got a little older he would smile at my ridiculous attempts to amuse him.

Harry proved to be more of a challenge. I had to take dozens of shots of him to get one or two decent images, and rarely would I be lucky enough to catch one of his smiles.

The first one I did capture was absolutely beautiful. He was lying propped up in his Moses basket, wearing a light blue Babygro and looking into the distance. The one eye he had was big and round like mine as opposed to almond-shaped like Oliver's and it was bright blue. His tilted smile just added to the charm of his beaming, unique face. When I printed the picture off, I cried. Back in Special Care I would never have dared to dream that I could take such a lovely photograph, let alone be excited to frame it and show it off.

Of course, not everyone knew Harry, and so there were times, painful times, when people would comment, stare or point. I found these days incredibly difficult. Preparing to take any baby, let alone twins, out is like planning a military operation, and so even a visit to Tesco required a lengthy preparation time before we left the house. We needed food and supplies like any other family, but my heart would thump in my chest. I would be gasping for breath and my hands would sweat and shake, clinging to the buggy as I pushed my boys through a sea of glances and whispers.

On one occasion, two boys followed me and the buggy around the store, facing me at the end of the tinned goods aisle so that they could have more time to stare at the boy with one eye as they whispered and giggled. It broke my heart.

I hated the twisted grimaces that people pulled when they saw Harry; the way they elbowed their friends to look, too; the pointing or the whispering behind raised hands. I would tell Mark, but often he hadn't seen it, which led me, years later, to the conclusion that maybe they were staring at us because I was staring first, willing their eyes to turn in our direction to justify my fears. Of course, there were times when people naturally noticed, but I do think now that I walked around with a heightened sense of awareness, wondering what everyone thought of my child and the terrible mother who had let him down. If I could go back in time and talk to myself now, this would be my best advice: don't go out in the world *expecting* it to hate and judge you or you'll find examples of where it does.

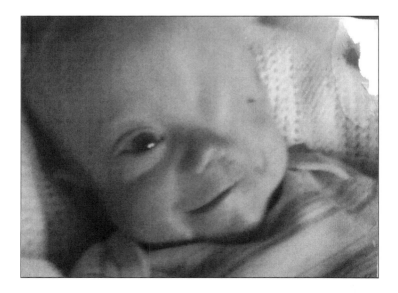

Learning to Adapt

By the end of 2005, we had a whole catalogue of professionals trying to help us find our way through the maze of challenges and decisions that were ahead of us. The visual impairment team gave us a book entitled *Learning to Look* – I remember flicking through the contents and thinking that 'looking' is never something that we consciously learn to do, we just do it. How many other things would require us to learn a glossary of terms?

The hearing impairment team provided literature on unilateral deafness; speech and language came with a how to guide on basic sign language. Sometimes I would sit for hours looking at the helpful information, but that's all I would do. I would stare at the black squiggles on the white pages which I knew my brain should be translating and processing as words, but it just wouldn't happen.

Occasionally I was struck with the unfairness of it all and wanted to stamp my feet, scream and thrown my hands up in the air like a spoilt child. However, I also remember still, calm moments of looking at the information and thinking, *we won't need to know this.*

Harry will be OK. We will be OK. Maybe I was a bit deluded or optimistic in those early days, but Harry has come so much further than anyone expected, and I think part of me – that quiet voice that often gets stamped on by the frenetic chaos of day to day thinking – always knew that he would.

Sometimes we would find a glimmer of hope in reports from the various tests which both boys had. One such moment was when the boys had their hearing tested at two months old. Oliver's hearing was statistically fine, as was Harry's hearing on his right side. The hearing level recorded on his left side reported that it was only slightly lower than the hearing found in typical babies, backing up the results of the MRI scan which showed normal inner ear structures. This was great news, but, just as with his optic nerve, it was bittersweet to think that he had come so close to having the hearing and the vision that his brother was enjoying.

Moments like this, when we were told that Harry had some 'normal' structures, gave us hope that, with some interventions and work on our part, he would be 'fixed'. I wince even as I type that word, but in the beginning we were looking at his catalogue of problems and trying to rank them in order of those which would cause him, and us, the hardest journey. In reality, there was no such list. In the medical world, even with the incredible advances in knowledge, technology and techniques, there are no short cuts or quick fixes for what Mother Nature omits, and the longer a child lives with their issues, the more adapting they need to do.

But adapt they can. While I struggled to cope with the visits, the reports, the advice, the facts, the decisions,

Harry was happily getting on with being all that he knew how to be – a baby. Blissfully unaware and unconcerned by his differences. I affectionately envied him for this at times, but my boy has since taught me well in the ways of 'loving who I am'. Sometimes I think I'm becoming as good at it as he has always been.

Our First Clinic

In October 2005 we made our first trip to Birmingham Children's Hospital. The room was large and hot, much like a sauna with less nudity. Sitting in a semi-circle facing us were about 15 people – 30 eyes all wearing matching 'don't be worried, we are here to help' expressions. If you have ever seen *Family Fortunes* where each family member is introduced to the host by the matriarch and repeats the same, "Hello, Bob", you'll have a pretty accurate idea of what the first couple of minutes in that clinic was like for us. We were introduced to everyone by the main consultant and told their names and job titles. I stopped trying to remember them all after number four on account of the fact that I could find them out at a later date if I needed to.

I was sweating and my heart was pounding as we sat there, our eyes moving from one person to the next while the other 28 eyes were firmly fixed on us and our boys, who were protesting in the double buggy. It felt like a job interview where I hadn't quite prepared enough. I was momentarily distracted from the introductions a couple of times by the low rumblings of voices: questions and opinions as the professionals talked to their neighbours and discretely gestured in Harry's direction. Exhibit B for the day on the conveyor belt of children who needed medical interventions.

The surgeons explained that Harry's condition was a very rare one (affecting between 1/3,500 and 1/26,000 live births in the UK – Wiki) not only in the fact that the umbrella term of 'Goldenhar syndrome' was diagnosed so infrequently, but that the ways in which Harry's face had been affected were at the extreme end of the spectrum. They stressed that he had many years of operations ahead of him to try and add some symmetry to his wonky face, and that his eye would be the first area of focus. There would also be operations on his nose, his ear and finally his jaw when his bones had grown fully. But they were 'for the future', we were told…out there in the distance where they could torment the moments when I realised that I loved my boy anyway and wished he could be accepted for who he was.

The surgeons explained that they would be consulting with other cranio-facial specialists in Australia, Japan and France to make the most of their expertise in deciding the best plan of action to create an eye socket for Harry. I am sure I was supposed to be impressed with this, but I wasn't. I just wanted to know that we were doing the right thing for our son and that he was in the best possible care – two questions that could only be answered with hindsight.

While one of the two main surgeons was talking, his partner was looking at Harry with curiosity and wonder. Taking in all the absent features; pressing on the fatty lump of skin above his nose; feeling his skull like some new age phrenologist. Of course Harry objected to all of this, and as a mother, my instinct was to snatch him to me. But I allowed him to be scrutinised as I knew that I had to. If we had left Harry as he was and never agreed to any surgery, we would have been depriving him of a chance of enjoying a life beyond the superficial judgements. A chance to be accepted and loved. And he, more than most, deserves those things.

There were times when I questioned my own motives. Was I secretly wanting Harry's disfigurements to be corrected so that I would have the child I had imagined? So that the wrongs I felt I must have done would be resolved? To ease my own anxiety when the stares and the questions appeared? So that my little family would be perfect and 'fit in'?

I would like to say no, but I do think that right at the start there was an element of truth in this. Knowing and loving my boys the way I do now, I feel terrible for even acknowledging this, but my intention is to explain every thought of an unexpected special needs mum, and sometimes, in the darkest moments, I did wish for a magic wand. But equally, it's important to recognise that those moments became fewer over time as I let go of the idea of what constituted a 'perfect' family and embraced the fact that I have two incredible boys who are actually perfect in their own right.

And so, we sat in the hospital with the psychologists making notes as we answered their questions (*Charlene – the mother – became emotional at one point*), the surgeons trying to prepare us in a ten-minute conversation for the start of our journey, and our boys getting frustrated and grizzly despite a regular administration of chocolate buttons. As we left, we both released huge sighs, knowing that in our uncertain and scary future, a path ahead was being laid.

Our Developing Boys

The health visitor came regularly and reviewed both boys. Oliver was gliding beautifully up the centre of the growth chart at the back of the health record, which stretched like a rainbow from the bottom left corner to the top right. Meanwhile, Harry was fighting to climb the same projection and was just below the lowest percentile. Reading the boys' health books now is like looking at the Premier League football table where two teams started in the same place but played their matches very differently. By the time the boys were seven months old, Oliver weighed 7lb 4oz and Harry weighed just 5lb 11oz.

The physiotherapist was also visiting and was pleased with Harry's progress in turning his head to the left. It was great to know that hours of encouraging Harry to track a glowing ball in the dark to stretch his left side neck muscles was paying off, but I didn't really feel that I was doing as much as I should. During one visit, as the physiotherapist commented that I was a good mum, I replied that I really thought I could do more.

She smiled and said, "You're doing more than many mothers I see with children like Harry."

In that moment I thought about all the times when people had said that Harry had come to us for a reason. I thought about all the moments that I had wanted to scream or hit out in response, but maybe there was some truth in it. And I felt glad that I could help Harry, and sad for the babies and the mums who were still lost.

It was moments like these when my love for Harry grew. Small, insignificant moments that together created a picture of me as a mum and Harry as my boy. I couldn't tell you the exact moment or time when I stopped feeling angry at our situation or stopped blaming myself, although I do know that this took years and I believe it underpins some of my big decisions for our lives. But alongside the anger were episodes like these when I got the approval I'd desperately sought as a girl – evidence that I could 'make things better' for us all – and times when I just sat and played with my boys. Talked to them and kissed them. Buried my face into their necks and sniffed their talcum-powdered fresh skin to make them chuckle. Times when I would look from Oliver to Harry and back again and see two cheeky little faces rather than a missing part of a jigsaw.

Although comparing them was often difficult, in some ways I was spurred on to encourage Harry through Oliver making progress, and advice that we were given to help Harry was also good for Oliver. The speech and language worker told us to talk to Harry about *everything* we were doing, and so, for example, we would talk to both boys about each and every body part as we bathed and dressed it. When I was teaching Oliver to speak, I would stick out my tongue and exaggerate the L in "I LLLLLLLLLove you", only to giggle as he stared intently at my tongue and copied. I would try it with Harry, too, hoping that even if he couldn't see my tongue well enough to copy it, he could at least hear my declaration.

We were unsure during his first year how much Harry could actually see. If we were close enough to him then he would gaze in our direction, but he didn't make or hold eye contact, and his one eye wobbled quite fiercely from left to right. In December we went to Great Ormond Street for tests that would inform the Birmingham team about Harry's vision. The hospital was enormous, even compared to Birmingham Hospital, and the corridors we walked down were narrow and quite old. People spilled from every room and milled around, clearly busy and focused. With the reputation that GOSH had, though, we felt sure that we were in good hands.

The bit of hair that Harry did have was scrubbed off with a rough pad, and plasters to hold the wires which would measure his brain activity were stuck to his scalp. He sat on Mark's knee in front of an enormous screen that showed a series of black and white moving images like a scene from a science fiction movie. Whatever was happening neurologically between his eye and his brain was being recorded and would be fed back to Birmingham. We only hoped that the data would be positive.

Back at Birmingham, the ophthalmologist made an appointment for us to see her. Before she told us the findings of the report, she completed some checks on Harry that looked very comical, including spinning around on an office chair with him on her knee so that she could see how fast his eye stabilised when they'd stopped. Then she handed him back to us.

The data had shown some brain activity which meant that Harry could definitely see some movement, but the consultant looked at us sternly as she said, "I think you should prepare yourself for the fact that Harry won't have much vision at all in his eye."

We were devastated. We were still adjusting to the idea of surgery to correct what was missing, but we'd thought that Harry was fortunate enough to have at least one functioning eye through which he could enjoy the world. Now we were being told that this had been taken from him, too.

I cried. Again, it all felt so cruel and unfair. How many more times would we be here, feeling cheated on Harry's behalf? We had no idea what, if anything, we could do to help him, and we were left feeling helpless and hopeless.

We sat quietly for a while, trying to digest the news. I was wondering how on earth I would explain yet another setback to our friends and family while delivering the positive slant that I was now working so hard to find in every situation.

Back to Work

The time was rapidly approaching for me to return to work at the primary school exclusion support centre that I had been setting up when I fell pregnant. My boss had agreed for me to return for three days a week to accommodate the numerous hospital appointments and visitors to the house that Harry required, and this felt like a great balance.

The prospect of work felt like a welcome break from the intensity of being at home. I'm not sure whether that's a special needs mum issue or an every mum issue. Certainly most of the mums I've spoken to since I had my boys enjoy the time when they can be an adult in their own right again. However, to return to work, even part-time, I had to find childcare for my boys. This was going to be no easy task.

We were keen to ask for recommendations from other parents, but Harry had additional needs that meant we had to pay close attention to the childcare settings as well as considering whether we believed the staff had the skills to care for him. It was clear that Harry needed something a little bit different. The room he was in needed to be well lit with natural light. We wanted him to have outside access, but didn't want an assault course of pots, benches and equipment that he would have to navigate with his limited vision. We also wanted him to have plenty of items to stimulate his senses rather than just amuse and entertain him.

Our wish list was looking like quite a challenge as we visited nursery after nursery, and we felt like Ofsted inspectors as we grilled the managers about the care they provided. Then we found Staffordshire Moorlands Children's Centre and our spirits lifted.

The baby room had half an entire wall of floor-to-ceiling windows and was flooded with natural daylight. The rooms were bright and inviting, and each child had their own cot for their afternoon naps which were separated from the play area by a safety gate. The area outside the patio doors was decked, and the only toys out there were the items that the children took with them, which meant that Harry could wander freely but safely within the confines of the wooden fences. The walls were covered with textures and concave/convex mirrors to reflect the images and intrigue the children, although Harry managed to create his own interest. The staff seemed lovely, and when we were shown the specific sensory room full of soft matting, fibre-optic lighting and bubble tubes, we were sold.

The only issue we had was that Harry required one-to-one care, but he was too young to go through the process of statutory assessment to determine whether the local authority would cover the costs of his education.

I was getting used to completing paperwork telling agencies that could provide financial support how crappy things were. They didn't want to know the success stories or the anecdotes of happy moments. The Disability Living Allowance form was a torturous process of recording, in black and white, everything that was difficult about each day and night. It required me to calculate the number of minutes that I spent feeding, washing and generally watching Harry within each 24-hour period. As he got older, this became more depressing as I prided myself on looking for the many positives in each day. However, the financial forms were less soul crushing, and tested my maths skills more than my emotions.

After much to-ing and fro-ing of forms and information, we were given financial support for Harry's one-to-one and 'wrap around' care outside of the hours for every child under the age of three which are paid for by the government. We were approaching new chapters in our lives now with excitement instead of apprehension. In February 2006, I returned to work and my babies – now little boys in a big world – started nursery.

Whatever the Future May Bring

Leaving the boys was hard at first. I'm sure every mother finds this, but Harry's needs were so complex and I was so familiar with reading his little distress or pleasure signals that I worried about how he, and the nursery staff, would cope.

I underestimated how well he would communicate with the staff, and how well they would understand and respond to him. Both boys flourished at the Children's Centre. I regularly had photographs of them showing me the activities they had been doing. Each day when I collected them, Oliver's little face would light up and he would crawl quickly towards me before climbing up my legs and being thrown onto my hip for kisses and cuddles. In time, Harry would recognise my voice, turn his head towards me and smile to acknowledge that Mummy had arrived. These were the moments that melted my heart and strengthened our bond.

In June 2006, Mark and I got married. As neither of us was religious we decided on a civil ceremony at a local hall where we also held the wedding breakfast and our evening reception. It was an incredible day, and we all enjoyed the glorious heatwave of that summer in spectacular surroundings.

As I took my wedding vows and said the line "Whatever the future may bring", I thought about Harry, his operations and the decisions ahead of us. In that moment, promising that Mark and I would be there for each other, I cried as the enormity of the future touched me lightly, like a fleeting reminder that it was waiting for me. I laughed it off and we continued to have an amazing day, but I vividly remember that a future that held so much uncertainty for us all momentarily overwhelmed me.

Exactly one week after we got married, we celebrated our boys' first birthday. I watched the clock from the early hours of the morning. At 6.30am, I relived the moment that our boys had arrived and I sobbed. This day should have been a celebration of the happiest day of my life – the day I'd had the babies that I had so proudly carried and been excited to meet. The day our future as a family unit started. Of course, this is exactly what did happen, but our family was far from the one I had expected and our future was careering through unfamiliar territory. On that first anniversary, I felt incredibly cheated. When 10.30am arrived – the time that Dr Mona had told us the news – I was almost crippled with physical sadness.

Thankfully, I had the birthday boys to coax me out of the darkness and plans to keep my thoughts otherwise occupied to make sure that they had a fantastic day. I arranged for a bouncy ball pit to be delivered to the house, and family and friends joined us for a birthday barbeque that afternoon as I played the part of efficient 'hostess with the mostest'. This pattern of distraction and repression years later would unravel the very person I was.

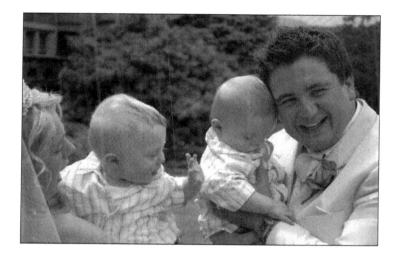

Harry Leads the Way

My boys were growing and developing as children do. I had expected Oliver to take the lead in hitting milestones and skills, so I was often surprised when he didn't. Shame on me!

I remember a few occasions when we were at Mark's parents' house with the boys in walkers, racing around the wooden floor. They would approach the French doors from the kitchen into the conservatory and Oliver would ram into the frame along the floor, protesting at the fact that he was stuck. Harry, however, would lift the sides of the walker up, much like a pantomime dame lifts her skirt, and place it on the other side of the frame. We were all astonished, but Harry, as always, was totally unaware of how much he'd impressed us.

Similarly, when we were teaching the boys how to crawl down the stairs, Oliver needed constant reminders and demonstrations. Harry was shown once or twice and mastered it without any problems. Whereas Oliver was a baby developing typically with the same awareness, depth perception and related trepidation that most babies have, Harry was not restricted by the idea that he may hurt himself and was determined not to be stopped when he had something on his mind. His tenacious spirit was, and still is, one of his greatest qualities, and I have watched him wrestle courageously with his frustrations and challenges over the years. Every day he makes me proud, as does Oliver – my treasured boys.

The year 2006 did not pass without its dramas, though. In February, Harry developed a rash. My first reaction was to try the 'glass test' and so I rolled a tumbler over the rash, which was rapidly spreading over his little body, expecting to see it pale below the pressure. When it didn't, my first thought was of meningitis.

Because Harry's breathing could at times be compromised by his restricted airway, we were on the 'open access' register at Macclesfield Hospital. This meant that we could bypass A&E and go straight to the children's ward, which is exactly what we did. Harry refused to allow the doctors to take blood from him, and it was incredibly painful watching him thrash about in so much distress, not being able to explain to him why it was all happening and reassure him that it would be fine. Eventually, the doctors were able to get enough blood to permit a test for the meningitis virus and we waited for what felt like an eternity for the results.

At times like this, it really didn't matter that he looked different, just that he was healthy. The thought that there could be something wrong with him frightened the life out of me. It was another of those moments when I knew that, despite the difficult days and the dark moments, I loved Harry just like I loved Oliver. There was no difference in my instincts to protect and nurture my boys. I think that moments like this helped me to put some perspective into my life.

I was so very relieved when the blood test results showed that Harry had a viral infection that required only antibiotics, but he had to stay in hospital for a few days while the antibiotics were flushed intravenously though his system. This meant time away from Oliver, and I had my first taste of being separated from one of my boys since they had come home. Being without either boy was difficult, and the anxiety was heightened because I was aware that I had been fighting my way through a fog in the early days when I should have been bonding with Oliver, and that every moment of his formative years was precious. Being away from Harry filled me with guilt and I panicked that something would happen to him if I wasn't there. Either way, I felt like I was losing.

The Balloon

We had visited Birmingham on a couple of occasions since our first meeting, once to discuss the clinical photographs and for the surgeons to update us with regard to the opinions and advice of their overseas colleagues. The second time was so they could tell us the plan for Harry's first major operation. A tiny balloon had been made in France. I imagined it to look like a small water balloon. The surgeons in Birmingham were going to try to insert it into the small gap that should have been Harry's eye socket. Although this gap was still closer to his temple than the bridge of his nose, they informed us that they hoped the inflation of the balloon would push the soft bones closer to its eventual destination, making later operations to expand the gap into an eye socket in the correct place much easier.

Attached to the back of the balloon would be a small tube which would lead to a 'reservoir' just under Harry's scalp. The soft, spongy lump would be the site of fortnightly injections of 0.5ml of saline solution which would work its way down the tube and slowly fill the balloon. It all seemed to make sense, but when I asked what would happen if it didn't work, the response stunned me.

The main surgeon said that the worst case scenario would be to leave Harry until he was older and then do a carpentry job on him. I had no words. I was processing that comment and what it meant for Harry's future. Either this operation would be a success and the first of several to reconstruct his face, or it would fail and Harry would have to wait until his bones had stopped growing, only to be hacked at like a piece of wood.

I am sure that the image I had in my head of random chopping and gouging was in no way what the surgeon had meant, but by the time I got to our car I was fuming. Crying, I rang Dr Mona and left a message with his secretary whom I was now on familiar terms with. She commented that she had never heard me so upset, and I presume that was why Dr Mona rang me back almost immediately.

I relayed the conversation to him through a frenzy of snot and tears. I told him that I wanted another opinion and for someone else to look at Harry's case. He was excellent at calming me in his deep, soothing voice with its foreign-tinged accent. He reassured me that Birmingham is an incredible centre for cranio-facial work, but unfortunately surgeons sometimes lack the people skills that doctors have due to the fact that most of the people they deal with are unconscious.

This made sense, and after Mark and I had talked it through, we decided to continue with the operation and trust that the surgeon's experience was better than his charisma. It is a decision that I now regret, but we truly believed that we were making the right decision for our son at the time.

*****

On 10 October 2006 Harry had his operation. Both Mark and I went down to the theatre with him. I held his little body close to me as the anaesthetists placed the mask over his face. He struggled against me, wriggling to be free from the mask and screaming in panic. Then, he just stopped. His body went limp and there was silence.

The team asked me to lay him on the bed, kiss him and leave, so I placed his tiny body on the huge adult bed, kissed his head through sobs and gasps, and we left. It was awful.

While he was in theatre, all thoughts other than *I hope he is OK* were suspended. The agonising wait seemed to last forever. We were unsure how long he would be in surgery, but almost three hours after kissing his head, we got the call to collect him from the recovery room. As we raced to be reunited with him, we literally bumped into the surgeons as they came out of the lift. They told us that they were thrilled with the operation and had already managed to inflate the balloon with 2ml of the saline solution, which gave the whole procedure a head start.

I have no words for how relieved we felt to know that it had been a success. In an instant, we felt like the future was full of possibilities again.

Harry's head had been wrapped in the style of a turban in layers and layers of bandage and a patch covered his left eye. His face looked swollen, and purple and dark blue bruising was already beginning to develop. He was sleeping, still affected by the anaesthetic, but we sat either side of his high cot and, dropping the bars at the side, held one of his hands each.

As much as I was thrilled to have him with us again and to be told that everything had gone to plan, a part of me was still sad that he was having to go through this at all. It didn't change anything and it certainly wasn't helpful, but at times I felt so angry that my son should have to go through so much.

The Hospital Mums

Harry stayed at Birmingham for a week, and I slept on a camp bed at his side on a ward full of other mothers and children who had undergone a variety of operations. I chatted with many of the mothers, and we swapped magazines and stories of how we had all ended up there. It was good to talk to other mothers who had children facing problems. I wonder whether it is natural to compare your own situation with others', but I found myself doing it anyway. On some occasions I felt that their children's problems were less severe than Harry's, but rather than envy their less complicated lives, I felt glad for them.

In contrast, there were parents for whom Birmingham was practically a second home. Here's my quick guide to spotting these mums.

They had friendly banter with the staff, having clearly been there long enough to know the people behind the uniforms. I still looked at name badges and started most sentences with, "Erm…excuse me…"

They helped themselves to the supplies and equipment that their children needed. I waited and tried to catch the eye of anyone in between their duties, feeling like a thief if I even attempted to help myself.

They were well trained in the methods of recording amounts of food and liquid consumed in folders which a novice mother like me dared not touch.

They had more home comforts than someone who was only staying for a week would ever need.

They were less paranoid about leaving their child in the care of the staff while they went to shower or eat, and would casually call to nurses that they were just nipping out. I didn't dare go to the toilet for fear of something happening in my absence.

The visitors who came to the bedside came to see the mother as much as the child, having got used to Mum being there so often.

They didn't jump out of their skin when the monitor alarms went off. In fact, I remember watching one woman reach up and knock her child's monitor on to mute while reading *Take a Break*. Meanwhile, I stared at the numbers on Harry's machines, trying to memorise and interpret them, and would have had a meltdown if one of the alarms had gone off. Thankfully, they didn't.

The selflessness and patience of these mothers amazed me. While I dreaded to think that I would ever have to experience such a long stay in hospital with Harry, I hoped that I would take it in my stride like them.

*****

Two days after his operation, Harry's bandages were slowly unpeeled, and we held our breath as we waited for his new face to be revealed. The slit of his preformed eyelids on the left side of his face was now much fuller and protruded from the previously sunken hollow space like the fleshy appearance of tiny lips. He certainly looked different, and as I looked at the little face that I loved, I hoped that Harry would have approved.

To access his eye socket, the surgeons had had to cut his skull open from one side to the other. Between where his two ears should have been ran a zigzag scar, each segment about two inches long. Someone having a bird's eye view of the top of Harry's head could easily have mistaken it for a Halloween pumpkin. While it looked like it should have been incredibly sore, Harry appeared to be relieved to have the bandages removed.

He was understandably grizzly after the anaesthetic, and though he slept well during the first night, he cried through the following four nights. Surrounded by other children and sleeping mums, I felt an insane amount of pressure to soothe him back to sleep. However, my frustration only exacerbated his anxiety, and so it was a long week of sleepless nights and slow days.

The surgeons were very pleased and confident that everything had gone to plan, and so we felt that it was worth it. Among the notes and scraps of paper on which I've recorded my thoughts or feelings over the years, I recently found the tatty A4 piece of paper on which I had written the day by day account of Harry's first operation. Two days after his surgery, I'd written: *The bandages have come off today, revealing a huge scar, but you have been laughing since Mr Weston took it off so you're obviously feeling better. You're playing in the cot at my bedside as I write this and I am very proud of you, my brave and beautiful boy.*

Oliver's Empathy

Oliver had attended nursery for his three usual days and my mum and nan collected him. Mum said that each afternoon he looked to the door expectantly as they walked in, only to look deflated when I wasn't there. He was missing me, and I was missing him.

I know that siblings of children who have life-limiting conditions often say that they feel the other child took priority. Although they understand as they grow why this is, I wish with all my heart that I could explain to Oliver just how hard it was for me to be apart from either of them.

Oliver is sensitive to my mood, and from a toddler he could read my body language well. When he went through the typical toddler stage of deciding whether cannibalism was for him and biting other children, I would arrive at nursery, sign the 'incident form' and squat down to his level, exaggerating my facial expressions and telling him how I was feeling. I did this when he had good days, too, and by the time he was two-and-a-half he could recognise and articulate emotions such as angry, disappointed, happy, and proud. Now, he is incredibly adept at reading my mood from the tone of a couple of words or the way I am breathing. His emotional intelligence is amazing and his empathy skills are better than some adults I know.

This does, however, leave him vulnerable to experiencing feelings more intensely. I sometimes wonder whether our separation during my stay in Birmingham was the start of an anxiety that came to grip and terrify Oliver as he grew older.

An Unenviable Task

In January of 2007, the surgeons continued to inflate the balloon. For the first few weeks, Harry, Mark and I travelled the 50-mile round trip to Birmingham so that 0.5ml of saline solution could be administered through the reservoir and into the balloon. This involved inserting a long, fine needle into the lumpy area just below Harry's scalp and pressing the syringe to flush the liquid through.

On the first few occasions, Mark sat Harry on his knee and held him as he screamed hysterically and struggled to get out of his grip. With nothing else to do but watch, I remember feeling extremely anxious and wondering, on several occasions, whether we should just abandon the procedure altogether and leave him in peace. However, I tried to think of the bigger picture – of a life for Harry where he was accepted and judged on his merits rather than his appearance alone. I hoped and prayed more than once that we were doing the right thing for him.

After a few visits, the surgeons suggested that they show us how to complete the procedure so that we could do it ourselves at home. This meant that I was now the one restraining Harry and Mark had the unenviable task of inserting the needle. It was a tense and stressful procedure, and although we got relatively quick at completing it over time, it never felt any easier. Harry would notice the signs: 'the bag' coming out of the cupboard and the dining chair being placed in the middle of the kitchen, and he would start to squeal, a high pitched distress call accompanied by shaking and sweating. Mark did much of the preparation out of Harry's sight and I would sit him on my knee, holding his arms down by his side with my right arm and his forehead against my right shoulder to steady his head.

In an impressively swift motion, Mark would clean the reservoir with the antibacterial wipe, insert the needle and depress the saline solution. I admired him each and every time for being the 'bad guy', although I think that Harry did hold it against me for being Mark's accomplice for quite some time too. What he lacks in aesthetic symmetry he makes up for in memory cells!

A Spanish Nightmare

In June my boys turned two years old. On their first birthday I had been gripped by the memory of their birth, but I had just married Mark and had organised their birthday party so I'd had plenty to prevent me from wallowing too much. This year, however, I had no such distractions. I was awake to see the pre-dawn haze again and thought about the night that I was in labour – all my fears of giving birth and the excitement of meeting my babies. Then, I recalled the chaotic moments when it was realised that Oliver's 'head' was actually his bum and that I would need an emergency caesarean. I watched the clock and painfully relived every moment as if it were happening again.

As I tickled them both and giggled with them, I knew that those early feelings should not matter. That they were nowhere near as important as where we were right at that moment – happy and coping. But the sadness lurked within me still, and on my boys' birthday, the day most mothers relive the moment they welcomed their child to the world, I felt it more keenly than at any other time.

A few months later, Mark and I decided that we needed a break and made plans to visit his parents' holiday house in Spain. It would be our first family holiday and we were as excited as we were apprehensive. The boys coped well on the flight and we were feeling positive as we landed in Spain and Mark went to collect the hire car. We loaded up the bags, the buggy, the car seats, the children and set off to the house.

The boys thoroughly enjoyed their time in Spain. There was both an indoor and an outdoor pool at the complex and so they happily splashed for hours in the glorious sunshine. We ventured to the beach twice, but the sand would get so hot that the boys were unable to set foot outside the circular shadow cast by the parasol. While we found this to be an effective deterrent from them running off, it also frustrated the boys and so generally we stayed around the house and the poolside.

Mark's parents had only recently bought the property and a few jobs still needed to be finished. One of them was the gate from the garden to the rest of the complex which had yet to be fitted. We were used to creating barricades at home and so we used bikes and benches and all sorts of summertime accessories to block the gateway. Although the area resembled a junk yard, we were satisfied that the wall was impenetrable for Harry.

One afternoon as I prepared lunch in the kitchen, I had an instant feeling that something was wrong. Harry and Oliver never chatted together; they played, but I was used to not hearing their antics. Yet I had a heavy, sick feeling that I hadn't experienced before.

Walking out into the garden, I saw Oliver happily playing beneath the child size chair and parasol set.

Mark was inside, but when I called to ask him if Harry was with him, I already knew the answer.

And then I knew what had happened.

Staring at the gateway, I noticed a small gap at the bottom where the frames of both bikes crossed but neither was low enough to block the hole completely. It was far too low and small to fit an adult through, but a determined and mischievous child could slide through on its stomach.

I frantically tore at the items in the gateway, screaming to Mark that Harry had gone. As I hurdled over the lowest objects, I stood paralysed by fear on the paved path. To my right was the car park, secure but still dangerous. To my left were networks of paths that led around the complex. At each junction where one path met another there was a low circular bed which contained a fountain, and Harry was fascinated by them, not to mention the swimming pool which he loved. I had to make a decision but was terrified that it would be the wrong one.

Three months earlier in Portugal, a three-year-old girl had disappeared from her bedroom while her parents were dining. The story of Madeleine McCann had gripped me, my friends and everyone as international police searched for her and her distraught parents appealed for help. Briefly, the case flashed through my mind as I decided to race to the swimming pool, holding my breath and feeling sick with adrenaline and dread.

He wasn't there.

Mark had run to the edge of the car park so as not to be too far away from Oliver, who was crying hysterically. Mark shouted to me that he couldn't see Harry, so I ran down the path which was parallel to the swimming pool, across the front of the house to the main entrance gate. On my left was a small park area with a few sit-on bouncing figures and a couple of swings. Harry was wandering aimlessly between them and humming *Twinkle, Twinkle, Little Star*.

A sob of relief escaped from me as I ran towards him and scooped him up into my arms. He giggled, totally unaware of how frantic we had been, and I walked back to the house clutching him as if he were a baby again. Oliver was still crying and needed reassuring, and so I passed happy Harry to Mark and sat on the grass to cuddle Oliver until he was calm. All of this had happened in only a couple of minutes, but it had felt like an eternity. If anything, it made us more aware of how cautious we had to be.

*****

Progress

Back at home, the boys were still enjoying their days at nursery, and I loved looking at the photographs that the staff sent home showing their activities: Harry wearing his lunch and grasping his fork in his fist; toys in a water tray and Harry's coy smile as his key worker tried to dip his hand into the tray; the boys walking along a path of paper with their feet covered in paint, tiny red and blue footsteps behind them. Their expressions of concern made me chuckle. So many moments captured of my boys doing the same activities.

I hoped that now Harry was socialising with other children, he would become more interactive with them and with Oliver, but by the end of the year he was still finding this difficult. He played with the same baby toy or toys for hours, sometimes days, and was mesmerised by their colours and noises. He would sit with the group to sing nursery rhymes, but then would choose to play alone again, albeit tolerating a few children beside him. He used the staff, and us, as 'tools' to acquire whatever object he wanted and didn't seem to be making particularly close bonds with anyone in the room, and yet everyone loved him. The children, never fazed by his clear disinterest in them, tried to engage him with their babble and their toys, and the staff were always clearly delighted to see both of my boys.

I was impressed that they tried so hard with Harry, until I realised that 'tried' implied a conscious effort on their part, when in fact they thought the world of my unresponsive and antisocial boy. That is the power of Harry, and many other special needs children for that matter. His unique habits and little ways and the mysterious, unspoken dance of a relationship that developed between him and those around him touched people in a way that typically developing children don't always manage. It took me a few years to see that 'special needs' also means gifted.

Both boys were developing beautifully in their own way and at their own rate at the nursery, but I couldn't help but notice that as they grew older, the gap in their abilities seemed to be widening. By the time the boys were 14 months old, Oliver knew several phrases, people's names and could imitate a few animal noises. Harry managed to say hi and used Mamma and Nanna, although not always correctly.

By the time the boys were 27 months old, Oliver was an unstoppable chatterbox. He was linking words, knew his colours and numbers, recognised and greeted various family members and was always singing. Harry had only added Dadda to his vocabulary. Oh, and screaming. This escalated in correlation with his developing understanding and related frustration. The older and bigger he became, the more fierce and physical his tantrums were, often resulting in him smacking himself in the head or throwing himself to the floor.

He would hand lead me to the area that he wanted (usually the biscuit cupboard) and point using my hand while grunting and making pleading noises. Often I would pick him up and get him a bit closer so that he could point to or touch whatever it was that he wanted, but if it was more complex than a simple choice, I would only end up calming his anxious state after several failed attempts. The minute he asked for something, I would have the 'fight or flight' adrenalin rush and almost feel against the clock to meet his needs to avoid him becoming distressed. Often we managed; sometimes we didn't, and we would all feel exhausted afterwards. On more than one occasion, both Mark and I agreed that if we could have changed anything instantly for Harry, it would have been to give him the gift of speech.

*****

In October 2007 I attended a core group review for Harry at nursery. Harry's key worker, nursery management, Angie our health visitor and Kate our social worker attended. I can't remember how we ended up having a social worker now. It's a bit like this: you get support from everywhere, accept it and then forget how it all came about in the first place.

We sat discussing Harry's slow but steady and positive progress as well as his continuing needs, which I felt to be around issues with his sleep patterns and speech and language. Kate commented that during the review she had conducted of Harry and us at home, I had said that I would like more input from speech and language and had considered paying for private therapy. This was true, but I wanted to make two things clear. Firstly, I was not saying that we were not satisfied with the great support Harry was already receiving, but we hoped to give Harry as much support as we could. Secondly, I was well aware that there was no speech and language (SAL) magic wand that could, in a matter of weeks, have Harry chatting away like Oliver.

Before I had finished my next sentence, heads began bobbing up and down and a chorus of 'mmmmmms' in agreement circled the room. I said that, after all, we didn't really know whether Harry's SAL difficulties were an indicator of more brain damage or delay. It wasn't easy, but I felt that I needed to ease the burden of politeness and allow everyone the chance to be frank. The relief that everyone felt once I had said that was tangible. No one had wanted to be the one to say, "But, Charlene, maybe it's his brain more than his speech. Maybe he will never get better." I felt quite empowered by this.

Then Kate summarised the key points made at the meeting and the home assessment. Although both meetings had been largely positive, I found myself staring blankly at the desk in front of me. Aside from Harry's infectious personality, cheeky smile and loveable qualities, I heard a shopping list of difficulties, obstacles and unknowns. My focus blurred briefly, then I felt Angie watching me so I blinked hard and fast, took a deep breath and smiled at everyone facing me. I imagine everyone saw through my masquerade of calm composure.

Kate said, "I think you are a very positive mum."

"I have my moments," I replied and swallowed an ache in my throat.

I Can't Fix This

The same week that I was reassured by Harry's steady progress, I was made to question my own.

At one of the primary schools I worked in, I had chatted a few weeks previously with a teaching assistant who had some experience of SAL strategies, and also had a son with dyspraxia. She told me about support groups as well as a local 'adventure playground' which was a great place for the children to play and mums to meet each other. The next week she told me about parent partnership – an organisation where parents could support each other and go on outings with other carers and siblings.

She smiled with her eyes – clearly a passionate advocate for the group – but I was mortified. In my mind I pictured myself squatting down in a corner of a room with my arms wrapped tightly over my head as if I were protecting myself from attack, and with this image came breathlessness and a heart that I could hear pounding in my ears.

I forced a smile and said, "It sounds good. Maybe in a while I'll try it, but – don't ask me why – I just don't feel ready for it yet."

She looked puzzled. Further conversation revealed that her son had been diagnosed aged nine, and as such, their journey had been very different from Harry's and mine. For her son, attending a disabled youth club had given him enough insight and knowledge of both the 'normal' and the 'special' children to decide for himself that being different was actually a good thing – much better than being one of the majority of children who were under pressure to conform to certain norms or standards which some would never achieve.

I wondered if that was true for Harry. Was I depriving him of a richer experience by not allowing him to mix with other disabled children and their mums? They might be able to understand and support me as well. Was I depriving myself? But I knew I wasn't quite ready. Part of me was still cowering in that corner.

I had felt that I'd been doing so well. I mentioned it to Mum, and as I talked through my thoughts, I stumbled across the realisation that yes, I had made progress in addressing my own feelings, but only within the comfort zone of my familiar world. I had introduced Harry to my friends, my places, my reality. While I had thought that would be enough, it suddenly dawned on me that not only had I not attempted to understand or join Harry inside his world, but the thought positively petrified me. I was fighting so hard to be a 'normal' mum, I didn't want friendships with other mothers based purely on our 'different' children. I didn't want to be a part of that community, yet my son was. Maybe this explained my struggle.

"There isn't a day when I don't wish he could have a life like Oliver – running around with his friends, chatting away and amusing everyone." Fat tears slowly rolled down my cheeks as I stared out of Mum's kitchen window at nothing in particular, feeling numb and empty. Mum put her arms around me for the millionth time and held me, while my brother, who hadn't seen me like this since the days of teenage hormones and dramas, watched in awkward discomfort.

"I can't fix this," I whispered over her shoulder. "I've always been able to sort things out and make them better, but I can't with this, can I?"

"No, sweetie," Mum replied, "but you can't carry on like this."

I wiped my face. Hearing the concern and wobble in her voice, I pulled away and smiled.

"I'm OK, honestly. Don't worry about me."

"But you're not! Stop doing this to yourself. Just let it all go," Mum begged.

"If I start," I said quietly, "I might never stop."

Oliver shouted from his baby seat at this point so I was back on autopilot. No time to stress. I kissed Mum and drove home, taking deep breaths.

At times I felt like a pressure cooker bubbling away with the lid on tight, yet at the same time I could feel almost detached from my own life. More than once, I saw new parents with twins, going about their day-to-day lives, and I would be frozen to the spot – rooted by an urge to watch what it must be like to enjoy the simplicity of life without disability. A life where hope and potential lay at the end of the sleepless nights. The life that I had wanted which now felt like the winning lottery ticket that had been ruined in the washing machine.

I could easily have been consumed by the oppression of self-pity and self-loathing, but I knew that my boys needed me so sense would return. I would carry on with my day without wishing the parents well in their lives. I took that with me, along with the snapshot of another world I would never know.

This is Harry

Dealing with my own emotions was difficult at times, but dealing with the feelings and reactions of other people was far more challenging. A lot of factors contribute to the sort of reaction that Harry receives. Generally, toddlers would notice Harry's face – or, more specifically, the absence of his left side – usually about the same time as he was wresting a toy away from them. They would first stare blankly and then cry.

One young child howled inconsolably, pointing blatantly at Harry while her mother balanced her on her hip, trying to fathom what on earth was wrong. As soon as she realised, she was mortified and ushered her daughter off. Some children, maybe early school age, would stare with their heads tilted and their curious gazes fixed intently on Harry as he wandered around, oblivious to their interest. Others would follow him as if hypnotised. Sometimes they would run off and grab their friends and a small group would form to take it in turns to watch the boy with one eye.

On one occasion I momentarily lost sight of Harry in the play barn. When I heard him whining, I saw him in the head lock of a much older child who was trying to prise his bad eye open. In a heartbeat, I had hurdled over the leather sofas and snaked my way through the obstacle course of tables and chairs like a whippet at Crufts. I snatched Harry from the clutches of the child and told him firmly that Harry didn't have an eye and that he wasn't to touch him. Meanwhile, Harry had already wandered off back to the baby section to play with more noisy toys.

At first, it was difficult for me to deal with these reactions. No one wants their child to be the source of tears, the thing of nightmares, the object of fascination, and so usually I would go over to an unconcerned Harry once the children had left him alone or the embarrassed parents had rushed them in the opposite direction. At those times, I would be so thankful that Harry didn't have the 'average intelligence and mental capacity' that we had hoped for him on the day of his birth. He was spared the hurt feelings that I so acutely experienced on his behalf.

We couldn't go anywhere without someone commenting, staring, pointing, whispering, or crying. At times I just wanted to stay at home, but my friend Caroline encouraged me (almost forced me) to go out with her support. We would visit play dens and barns and try to live a life I could so easily have hidden away from. For a long time, my heart would bang in my chest as we went into places and I would be scanning the room to find people who had noticed Harry. I imagine for most parents like me, the intensity of this anxiety lessens on its own, almost without them realising. However, I can tell you specifically the moment that it changed for me.

I was wandering around Mothercare with the boys in their buggy, hunting for a gift for a friend's new baby. I was focused on my search, yet acutely aware of the familiar signs that Harry had attracted his usual interest. A child was following us around the store as if we were playing a game of follow the leader. Within a few minutes, they had disappeared only to return with two other children. Now I felt like the Pied Piper as they followed us around the store, whispering and looking concerned as they tried to catch a glimpse of Harry.

As usual, I was feeling incredibly uncomfortable at this point. I was unsure whether to abandon my shopping mission and flee to the safety of the car, snarl discreetly at the children like a guard dog in the hope that it would deter them, or just carry on and ignore them. I remember, in the midst of my despair, thinking, *I can't keep doing this*, stopping the buggy and turning it around to face them, feeling all the while like I could be sick.

They stopped dead at the safe distance from which they had been following us.

"This is Harry," I said.

All of the children approached us then and squatted at the side of the buggy. One girl gently touched Harry's hand as if he might break, but he returned the gesture with a firm grip as if to prove that he was not a fragile mystery.

The brief conversation that followed went something like:

"Where is his eye?"

"He was only born with one."

"Why was he only born with one eye?"

"We're not sure. Sometimes things like this just happen and the doctors don't really know."

"Does it hurt him?"

"No. He's very brave."

"Will he get a new eye?"

"One day, yes. The doctors will make him a new eye so that he can look just like you and his brother."

"Oh. OK."

And just like that, they left us.

I was speechless. I'd suffered months and months of anxiety, intense surveillance of the children around us and fear, when all I had needed to do was to allow the children to meet the 'boy with one eye', know his name and realise that he was in fact very cute. I can't begin to tell you the power of that moment: the relief and the elation. It was like finding the simple answer to a question that had tormented and twisted the very heart of me for such a long time. I could breathe again, deeply and fully.

I continued shopping, but I knew right there that something had changed in me forever. The little voice inside had known I couldn't take much more and had somehow compelled me to stop. I felt so proud of myself for standing up for Harry and dispelling the curiosity rather than standing by until the fascinated spectators left, like the pathetic excuse for a mother that I had previously felt I was.

As time passed, I became confident in not only answering any questions, but also pre-empting those moments when a startled child may need an introduction to Harry, or a flustered parent may need reassuring after apologising profusely for their child's interrogation. It was perfectly normal for children to ask about Harry; in fact, it was much easier that way.

Often, I would thank children who came with insightful questions and, once they knew the answers, would fuss him and play with him, even though he didn't particularly welcome their friendship. I don't think it's any surprise that now, having dealt with the questions for years, I rarely notice people looking.

Not so long ago, I took the boys with my nan to a local park. We played on the equipment, and I introduced Harry to the children who wanted to know him and answered their questions. Hilariously, one little girl asked me to remove my sunglasses so that she could check whether I had one or two eyes. Some children are fantastic!

Later, a mother timidly broached the subject of Harry's syndrome. I explained the facts as I knew them and how Harry was affected, and equally unaffected, by his issues.

She looked at me with such kindness and said, "I've watched them all staring and whispering. It must do your head in. I think you're really brave and your little boy is lovely."

I have to admit that I was a bit taken aback by her admiration, not just because she was the first stranger ever to say something like that to me, but because I hadn't noticed, until she pointed it out, that people were indeed staring at us. The glances and the whispers behind hands were there, just as they always had been, but I hadn't even noticed them.

Times like this confirmed to me that the issues I had felt, the crushing sadness that had consumed my waking days and restless nights, weren't really to do with Harry's syndrome. Actually, they were about the ways in which

I had internalised his issues as a reflection on me as a person, and the ways in which I did and did not cope. That one moment in Mothercare changed the course of my life as a person and as a mother.

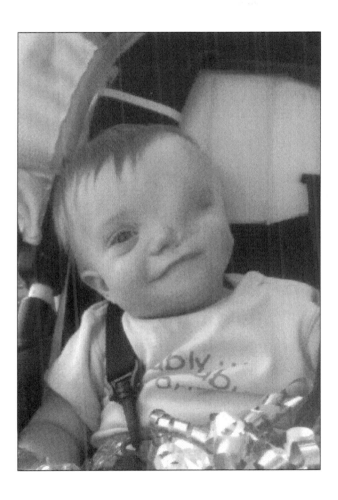

Never Give Up On Yourself

As well as me, Harry was making progress, too. In December 2007, the visual impairment team withdrew their support, saying that they believed Harry was only benefitting from the one-to-one attention and had acquired all the vision that he would need. Despite only having one eye, Harry coped fantastically well with all aspects of looking and discrimination, and I rarely even thought of him as being visually impaired.

I was so proud of him. I remember saying to his VI worker that I truly felt that I was in a place where I was able to celebrate his differences, and I wondered if Mark felt the same. For some reason, we rarely discussed our own opinions and feelings about what was happening. Although we would debate at length any options we had for surgery or interventions, our personal battles with the life we were still adjusting to sat between us like an elephant in the room.

In January, Harry moved into the next room at his nursery. As I dropped the boys off on the Monday morning, I was told that his previous key worker had been ill and so none of his information had been passed on to the new staff. I had fewer than five minutes to tell them all about my boy.

I panicked. All I could think to stress to them was the sign he used for 'more'. I didn't think to mention that they must approach him from his right side, or that he enjoyed music if he got upset. I didn't tell them that he responded better to varied intonation of voice, and so 'singing' an instruction to him worked better than just saying it. Or that he needed his food to be cut up into manageable-sized chunks for him to pick up.

As I drove away, I started to cry and soon had to pull over in floods of tears. I desperately wanted to be a good mum for my boys, but at the same time, I wanted to be successful as a person. I wondered whether to give up on my plans for teacher training and find work in a position with less responsibility which I could leave at a moment's notice. I don't actually believe that such jobs exist, but when you're in a state of panic, you invent all sorts.

When I was calmer I resolved that, while I could, I should follow my plan and face each challenge as I came across it. As much as it is not in me to give up on Harry, I knew that I couldn't give up on myself either. It felt selfish to want something for myself and not be driven solely by motherhood, but I firmly believe that a happy woman makes a good mother, and I desperately needed to be both.

A phone call later to the nursery confirmed what I should have known all along: Harry was fine and making his needs known quite well, even without my help.

Oliver's World

During the February half term, Caroline once again encouraged me to take the boys out to a play area in Holmes Chapel with her and her children. It was fantastic not to experience the usual anxiety about people's reactions to Harry, and I watched him proudly as he sat on a raised cushioned star in the middle of the ball pool, laughing to himself. I enjoyed the moments of peace while I knew where he was.

Oliver, on the other hand, was having a clingy day. Since I had been away from him during Harry's first operation, Oliver had become quite anxious and wanted me constantly at his side, particularly after Harry's Houdini episode in Spain. If I wasn't with him, he would often throw himself onto the floor, screaming and crying. This was generally simple enough to manage and entertaining Oliver was easy.

However, the balance shifted as soon as Harry started to walk around. In the play area, he would go from table to table, grabbing people's food and drinks. On one occasion he stood on a new-born baby in its car seat on the floor to reach a toy. No one was safe from his determined missions. Several times per visit, he would grab the hand of a stranger and drag them to play areas that he wanted to explore, or to the exit and the fresh air which he enjoyed so much.

As soon as I saw Harry doing any of these things, I became instantly torn between him and Oliver, who wanted my undivided attention. Harry couldn't care less where I was, but for this very reason, he was incredibly vulnerable, and at times a danger to himself.

During our half term visit to the play area, I found myself in such a position. I was watching and cheering Oliver down the slide as the emergency alarm sounded. I knew instantly that it was Harry and ran to the fire door at the side of the building. Sure enough, he had pushed the door open and was happily bouncing on his toes, flapping his arms and laughing hysterically at the noise and instant chaos that ensued.

I was back with Oliver within a couple of minutes, but that was long enough for him to disintegrate into a pile of tears and snot. I tried to console him while Harry wriggled in my grip, wanting to set the alarm off again, but Oliver was hysterical. For the first time ever, I felt unfairly furious with him.

What I didn't understand then was that Oliver in many ways had the worst of two worlds. He didn't have the brother or friend that he would have had if Harry had been a 'typical' twin, but equally, he wasn't an only child who had all of his parents' attention. As well as this, he never had the security of knowing that Mummy would be in one place all the time – the safe base from which he could explore his surroundings and return for regular top-ups of nose wipes, kisses and cuddles. Sometimes he would turn and I would wave and blow a kiss, but the next minute I could be rescuing a stranger who was being dragged around by Harry. Then Oliver would turn only to see an empty chair. No wonder he was so anxious.

As the boys ate their lunch, Caroline sensed my frustration.

"Be careful not to blame Oliver for being normal. It's not his fault."

She touched my hand and I cried. She was correct, of course. That's what I was doing, but I didn't fully understand until many years later. Not only was Oliver being unfairly burdened with the hopes and expectations I'd had for both of my babies, but I expected my precious toddler's developing ego and sense of self to be able to understand that I needed to protect Harry from his own curiosity.

I thought about it all the way home. I knew that I loved my boys with all of my heart, but the things I did, the words I said and the cuddles I gave needed to demonstrate this tenfold to Oliver. When we got home, my nan played with Harry while I cuddled Oliver and watched TV with him. We chatted and giggled, and I felt so very guilty as I looked at my little boy, perfect in every way yet perfectly lost at times in his own life.

I called Mark at work to say, "I take them out all the time. I answer children's questions about Harry's face and I split myself between them, but today was the day when I couldn't quite manage."

He told me that I was doing a great job, particularly as I was with them so much more than he was, and that he probably couldn't cope all of the time either. I was thankful that he supported my efforts and acknowledged how hard it was at times, but somehow, his words just added to the feelings of isolation which were creeping up on me like a long shadow on a sunny day.

*****

We both tried hard to keep life as normal as possible for Oliver. He had the most incredible mind: inquisitive and enthusiastic about everything. One Sunday we took both boys to the Blue Planet aquarium to explore life under the sea. Oliver was amazed. He walked around with his eyes as wide as saucers and his mouth agape with wonder. He marvelled at the colourful fish and sea creatures, and squealed with delight as he tentatively dipped his fingers into the rock pool, only to touch something in there and pull his hand out rapidly, throwing his head back and giggling. He pointed at anything that moved and asked question after question. We read the short posters to him and he listened as he watched the creatures they described. For years, he remembered many of the facts he heard on that day.

In stark contrast, Harry was unimpressed to say the least. He was not interested or even distracted by the creatures and colours darting past him. He was distressed by the crowds and disliked the heat of a confined area. He didn't want to walk, but he protested against being carried, wriggling and kicking out when we tried.

Oliver was mesmerised by the enormous glass wall behind which the sharks swam and he sat cross-legged to listen to the Sea Life staff tell their shark tales. Harry screamed. He didn't want to sit down. He didn't want to stand. Mark and I spent the day passing him between us, sweating and puffing as we wrestled with him while smiling and laughing as we joined Oliver in his excitement and fascination.

Mark sat with Oliver to watch the shark show and I went to the back of the room to cuddle Harry in a quiet spot. He didn't want to be cuddled. He wanted to sit on my legs, facing away from me, and rock backwards and forwards. He wanted his inner turmoil to have an escape, and ferocious rocking was it, followed by throwing himself back and splitting my lip.

Times like that were so hard, not because of having to manage Harry's behaviour, but because we both felt that Oliver missed out on sharing experiences with both parents. We visited the gift shop and then headed home. Oliver was asleep in no time, cuddling his Nemo accessories. Harry was asleep shortly afterwards, exhausted by the whole experience. We both knew how he felt.

There's a 'But'...

Over lunch one day at work, I read a text from a friend who was pregnant. I smiled as I read *It's a boy*, and then I read *but* and my heart sank. I remembered my TAMBA message – *Introducing Oliver and Harry...there's a 'but', though* – and felt sick.

I read the message slowly. *Cysts on his head; enlarged kidneys; I will speak to you all when I've stopped crying.* I wanted to cry myself. My lovely friend; her lovely family; her innocent son.

I replied saying that I was thinking of her, and then felt awful that I had forgotten to congratulate her on adding a boy to her family. The prospect of a child with problems totally eclipsed the fact that any child is a blessing.

She was on my mind all day, and that evening I texted to say that I was thinking of her. When she replied, *He'll still be our beautiful boy. You are my inspiration*, I was speechless. As I nursed Harry to sleep in my arms, I wondered if she really believed that or if she was saying what was expected, showing the strength of a mother while she contemplated an uncertain future like I had done.

I laid Harry down on his bed and stroked his head. As I watched him, I remembered asking myself if I would ever truly think of him as my beautiful boy when, in the early days, his differences were all that I saw. Now I felt awful. Here was my boy whom I loved with every breath of life in my body. I cried as I thought of my friend's journey. I hoped that the doctors were just being cautious and that her son would be fine. If they weren't and further problems were confirmed, she was in for one hell of a rollercoaster ride. I wished that I could prevent that for her, and for the first time I got an understanding of the total helplessness that my family and friends must have experienced. How awful it must have been for them to watch me fumble and stumble through the maze of hormones, grief and guilt in those early days. They were unable to help, only watch like hopeless spectators.

As I kissed Harry on his delicate little lips and whispered, "Love you," he grabbed at my finger, half-awake, half asleep, and squeezed it the same tender way he had done the first time I saw him lying in his incubator. For a long time, I had wondered if I would ever feel that overwhelming love or be able to forgive myself, and now I knew that my gorgeous, wise, ancient soul of an infant had always loved and never blamed me.

I waited until he had settled and tears filled my eyes again. I thought of my friend and my journey. I feared for her, yet I knew she would be OK. I was lost in her worry and desperation, yet I felt a quiet satisfaction that whatever the future held for her and her son, she would cope. Eventually she would enjoy and excel in the situation until it was time for her to be an inspiration to another mother.

Our Son is Not a Guinea Pig!

Since Harry's first operation in 2006, Mark and I had religiously been injecting the reservoir in Harry's head with saline solution once a fortnight. It never got any easier. If anything, Harry was becoming distressed sooner as he recognised even the early signs of preparation, but we persevered.

In March, Harry had an examination under anaesthetic to assess the inflation of the balloon and the development of the eye socket. A visiting expert surgeon from Japan and two further consultants from the Queen Elizabeth Hospital were present along with Harry's surgeon during the procedure to offer their opinions. We were assured that our efforts were worthwhile and returned in May of 2008 to discuss the next steps in Harry's reconstruction.

When we entered the clinic of professionals, which had once, long ago, been a daunting and intimidating experience, it somehow felt that we weren't the ones who were nervous. Their news wasn't good: the operation had failed. Although the balloon had filled with the saline we had inserted, it had not inflated in the direction that the surgeons had hoped. So now, instead of the start of a socket somewhere closer to its eventual destination, Harry had a larger hole which was still too close to his temple to be reconstructed into a socket.

We had been inflating the balloon for over a year. We had held our son down and fought back our own tears as he had screamed and thrashed about. Each visit to the hospital had required more CT scans, all of which we had been assured looked good. There had been optimistic talks of 'next steps' and we had held hope in our hearts. Now it had been removed, thrown to the ground and trampled all over.

I questioned why we had been told for so long that all was going well. Why were we only being told now that the procedure hadn't worked? Through the red mist of pure fury, I seem to remember hearing some attempt at an apology and an explanation that the professionals had tried their best to work with what was a very unusual case. We were assured that the balloon could be left in situ without causing any harm, therefore preventing any more unnecessary anaesthetics for Harry, but this was small comfort. We had trusted these people, their advice. We had followed their plan. Although I realise that sometimes it is difficult to predict the reaction of living human cells and organs when medical science intervenes, I blamed them anyway.

We were both distraught and not even back to square one. Harry now had scar tissue across his scalp which would never respond to further interventions in the way that healthy tissue does, a large hole in the side of his skull, and was petrified of any medical building, nurse or doctor. We were so far beyond square one that we didn't know what to do next.

The surgeons talked about other options but I wasn't listening.

"No, you've admitted yourselves that you can't predict what will happen if he has more operations. He's nothing more than a guinea pig to you, but he's our son!"

With that we left. We were devastated. We had placed Harry's health in the surgeons' hands and trusted that they would know the answers. Now we didn't know whom to trust or what to do next.

As angry as I was at the surgeons, I blamed myself more. It had been *our* decision to allow Harry to have the procedure and trust that it would work. Of course, if it had gone well then we would have never doubted ourselves, but now I wondered if I would ever be able to make another decision for him again. The one thing I did know for sure was that it would not be at Birmingham, and so we contacted Alder Hey Hospital in Liverpool and requested a second opinion, hoping with every fibre of our beings that we wouldn't be going through this again.

School Time

I am sure that Harry must have been incredibly relieved not to have to endure any more injections, and both boys continued to enjoy nursery. Although Harry pushed Oliver away whenever he attempted to play with him, I loved them being together every day. I hoped that somehow Harry would find a way free from his isolation and experience some enjoyment in the company of other children rather than the musical and visually stimulating toys which he played with repetitively.

His language was still incredibly delayed. He wasn't using gestures or eye contact, and turn-taking was non-existent. He clearly understood the words we used as part of his daily routine like 'dinner time' and 'bath time', but the few words that he had were limited. He preferred to hand lead adults to get whatever he required. Sign language had been unsuccessful with him, although I didn't know why. Maybe we gave up too soon. Maybe the articulate genius trapped within my boy felt insulted and patronised and was on the verge of amazing us all. I lived in hope and self-imposed torture.

In many ways, Harry had the independence and self-help skills of a toddler. At almost three years old, he still wore nappies and was unaware of his own body's signals that he needed to use the toilet. He needed food to be loaded onto his fork or spoon at meal times, although he would soon become annoyed with this and resort to using his fingers to feed himself instead, often ramming chunks of food into his mouth and choking. He was unable to dress himself at all.

However, he was making progress, and it was the small but important steps that I would focus on and celebrate. Whereas Harry had once thrown his plate and cup when he had finished or tired of them, he was now placing them onto the table carefully. Getting him dressed wasn't quite the battle it had been when we'd had to peel him out of his pyjamas. Instead he would hold his arms and legs out, a willing recipient of his daily outfit. And, although he still played alone during the day, the nursery staff offered me a brief moment of hope when they told me that he had approached a crying child one morning, furrowed his brow and tilted his head to one side. I dared to hope for just a moment that somewhere inside my boy's undiscovered mind he was wondering why this child was crying and what he should do about it. In fact, it was equally likely that he was wondering where the new noise was coming from and where the batteries went.

It might not have been the progress that the educational psychologists and the therapists were waiting for, but it showed me that some part of my boy was changing – responding differently. At a physiological level, surely this meant that there was hope for the complex wiring of his brain. At a social level, if he could approach a child, then maybe one day he would play with a child. I dared to hope that he might even make a friend. As helpless as I felt at times, I believed that Harry was merely a bud waiting to bloom in his own time. But it was all a guessing and waiting game.

Whereas in the early days I had struggled to see beyond Harry's condition, as his personality developed and my love for him grew, it saddened me to see the reports highlighting only his deficits. His severely disordered play and attention skills; his receptive and expressive language difficulties; his disordered interaction skills; his total lack of independence around feeding. It all read so bleakly, and yet I knew that my boy was so much more than any report could ever encapsulate. Though I knew that the assessment of his progress was judged against a 'typical norm', I also knew that Harry was far from the 'ordinary' population in a frustratingly magical way.

As the Local Education Authority gathered its reports on Harry and his needs, Mark and I were beginning to consider his options for school. My boys had attended nursery together for over two years by this time and I had enjoyed the routines of dropping them off and collecting them, knowing that they were together and happy. I wanted this to continue, and it was easier for me to think of my boys going to school together than it was to contemplate splitting them up and sending Harry to a special school. I had no idea what a special school would be like, but I imagined an institutionalised atmosphere of rules and routines and little creativity or spontaneity which may upset the delicate balance of the emotions of children like Harry. I still clung to the hope that Harry would cope with mainstream school and mainstream life – friends, homework, birthday parties, quarrels, awards – but that was unfair. Again, I was imposing my own hopes for his future and not considering his needs.

So we decided to visit a few schools to help us to decide. We knew which school we wanted Oliver to attend and we took both boys for a visit. It was, as most schools are, ordinary. The usual hustle and bustle of children and staff, displays showing the work of little hands and a playground full of equipment and coloured floor markings for games with friends. Oliver seemed to like it. Harry was oblivious to anything but the challenge of running away from us in the hunt for toys.

The head teacher picked him up and confidently slung him onto her hip as only a seasoned grandmother can, and we continued on the tour. Back in her office, we all agreed that Oliver would be fine here and felt excited for him, as well as saddened to think that our baby was ready for the next transition in a life that was racing by. There was a question mark over Harry, though. Although the head teacher spoke kindly about options for support in mainstream schools, her forced smile and gentle tone made me doubt that Harry would settle in quite as easily as his brother.

Special schools next. We only took Harry with us as we looked at alternatives to mainstream provision. I felt sick even before we arrived anywhere. This felt like we were admitting defeat, resigned to the fact that he would never enjoy the life that Oliver was taking for granted. I didn't want it to be true, and I hoped that we would be better off hedging our bets with Harry in a mainstream school with a one-to-one keyworker.

Both schools that we visited were 10 miles away in the rural town of Leek, Staffordshire. As much as I was impressed by the abundance of nature and rolling countryside, I felt that it was a long way from home for a little boy.

The first school catered for the needs of children with physical disabilities and offered a Conductive Education programme, which I had never heard of before but found fascinating. All the staff were trained to work with the child's own strengths and personality, essentially training them to control their own movements through cognitive awareness and consideration of their options and actions, thus encouraging the children to become active participants in their world. I liked the idea that each child's education was tailored to their own personality and needs, and as we wandered around with the head teacher, it became clear that the children were happy. The staff were experts in knowing not only the conditions they were supporting, but also the children for whom they cared.

Harry was his curious self and dashed from room to room, hunting for anything noisy and flashing to play with. As he dashed, oblivious to the things and people around him, he become an unwitting danger to the physically disabled children who were receiving their physiotherapy on the floors and benches.

I scooped him up into my arms to continue our tour, but as we walked through the school I began to feel uneasy. The children here were mainly immobile or extremely limited in their motor skills. Few of the children spoke, making groaning and long drawn out moans instead in their attempts to communicate, and the children who had enough motor control to look at us were impassive. I had no doubt that they were in the very best hands for them. From time to time I heard hearty chuckles and witnessed a communication that had developed between the staff and children that did not require formal language.

I was impressed, but I wanted to cry. Harry did not belong here. He was too mobile and too responsive for us to consider sending him to a school where he would differ from the other pupils as much as he would if he attended school with Oliver. As we walked to the car, I hugged him in my arms, kissed his little head and told him that I was sorry. I still don't really know what I was sorry for.

We felt exhausted, deflated and hopeless after the visit, but we still had the other school to see. We decided that we should get it out of the way before returning home.

Springfield School catered for children with moderate to severe learning difficulties and communication difficulties. Some were on the Autistic Spectrum. The staff, just as at the previous school, were clearly highly trained and skilled in working with the children. They welcomed Harry as he raced into their classrooms, ransacking boxes and tables in his furious hunt, as if they had known him for years.

The head teacher took us around the school and showed us the different rooms, their activities and a brief background on the needs that the staff were working hard to meet. In complete contrast to the image I'd had in my mind of a special school, this one was bright and inviting. Children were taking part in all manner of tasks, and I could see visual timetables and self-monitoring tools dotted around the rooms as they were encouraged to become as independent as possible. There were photographs of class trips into the local town to buy items and talk to the elderly residents at an old people's home. All of the visits had curriculum links, but more importantly, they provided an opportunity for the children to participate in the world around them.

As I realised that I liked it, I became a bit emotional. I think the head teacher assumed that I was struggling on the tour, but rather than hit me with the sales pitch to convince me that this was the school for Harry, she simply put her hand on my shoulder.

"I know that no parent ever *wants* to send their child to us," she said. "It's never a parent's wish to have a child with difficulties, but we try our best to make sure that they are happy during their time with us, and you would be welcome to come and see what goes on here anytime."

I was sold. Even now, thinking of how refreshing her honesty and sincerity were, I find myself moved to tears. My boy had to go to school eventually. Having seen Springfield, I felt wrong even to have considered mainstream school, and I knew that if I had to trust him anywhere and in the care of anyone, it would be there.

Crafty Boy

By the time Harry's second Early Years review was conducted in October, it was clear that he had made some progress not only in terms of his learning, but also in the development of his own unique personality. He was stubborn. At times, he would not respond to instructions or requests, but both Mark and I, and the nursery staff, knew better than to assume this was because he only had one ear. He would attend to the things that interested him and choose to ignore anything which didn't. I found it amusing when he plugged his ear with his finger and tilted his head away in order to 'block out' whatever he didn't fancy listening to – I'm sure we'd all love to be able to get away with that one from time to time.

When he was tested for his vision, the report stated that *Harry was shown three picture cards and was asked to select specific cards one at a time. He did not respond to this task. However, when different coloured Smarties were placed onto squares the same colour as the Smarties, Harry was able to see them and pick them up off the squares.* I laughed as I read this and guessed that he would have eaten the Smarties even before the people testing him could tick the 'able to discriminate between same coloured object and background' box. Clever, crafty boy.

He was also determined. Sometimes this was directed towards completing something that he did want to do, but often it was aimed at avoiding anything that he didn't. Meal times were a particular challenge and required Harry being put back on his chair dozens of times. The more frustrated I became, the more he ran, laughing as he went. Sometimes I would laugh at him, but at other times I would lose my temper and become very cross with him. It's no surprise that my reaction often correlated with the amount of sleep he had allowed me to have on the previous night.

Towards the end of the year, Harry started to sit beside other children. The staff in his room had been restricting the amount of time that he spent playing with the baby toys, and although he still did not interact with his roommates, he tolerated them being close to him without trying to push them away, and now actively sought comfort or help from staff members. They were only small steps, slight developments in Harry's ways and personality, but it was all moving in the right direction and I was feeling positive about his future.

I had also taken steps to improve my own future and had started the Graduate Teacher Training Programme with a view to teaching primary school children. It was physically and emotionally demanding, and maybe it wasn't the best timing when I was only getting about five hours of broken sleep with the boys, but when I get an idea in my head – a plan or a project – I'm all or nothing. So I threw myself into my training in the hope that I would be contributing to a brighter and more comfortable future for my family, as well as personally achieving some success and regaining the self-belief and pride which I had lost years earlier.

A Second Opinion

In November we received the appointment for our second opinion at Alder Hey Children's Hospital in Liverpool. By this time, we were used to walking into the meetings known as 'clinic' to be greeted by a sea of eyes and smiles. Alder Hey was no different.

Their plan, the consultants told us, was to admit Harry over a couple of days, during which time they would run their own MRI and CT scans as well as speech and language, palate, bowel and sleep investigations, and medical photographs. We were used to hearing that Harry's was a unique case and that we should bear this in mind when considering what options were available to him, but the consultants were now talking much more positively about how many options were actually available.

Their optimism was infectious. We still questioned whether transferring Harry's care was the right thing to do in our situation, but we decided not to make any decisions until after the investigations had been conducted and the Alder Hey consultants had a more definite plan. After all, we had misplaced hope before, and so this time it felt even more crucial to get it right.

Harry and I stayed in Alder Hey for three days in January 2009, during which time he was poked, prodded, scrutinised and assessed. In March we returned for the professional verdict on the various possibilities for the future of our boy, and it all sounded good. Unlike previous clinics, Mark and I were involved in discussing the options available, and each was presented with the associated pros and cons.

Of course, at this stage, there were not any big decisions to consider, but it was comforting to know that our opinions were as much a driving force in Harry's future as those of the medical team. We discussed the various methods of creating an eye socket and prosthetic eye, and then, for the first time, we were given an insight into the surgery which would follow this – Harry's nostril, his ear and his jaw. This would take us into Harry's late teenage years, which felt like a long time away back then. But for the first time, we had a timeline, albeit sketchy, of what lay before us all. Even a rough plan, an idea of a future, was less terrifying than the unknown and the guessing games which we had been playing for so long.

The lead consultant was keen to make it clear that Mark and I would have the final say about Harry's procedures – "After all, he's your boy" – and so we transferred Harry's care to the team at Alder Hey and placed his life in their hands.

*****

That spring saw another change for Harry. Unlike Oliver, who had to wait until the autumn to start school, Harry joined Springfield a term and a half early to allow him more time to settle in. I had no doubt that Harry was going to be attending the very best setting for him and so I didn't feel too concerned about his first day as a 'big boy' at school.

Getting him there, however, was a different matter. The local authority provided transport for the children who lived in our town and attended Springfield School, and to my surprise there were quite a few. So on his first morning of school, my boy – still wearing his infant-sized clothes and looking like a Borrower off on an adventure – boarded the 'special bus', as I and countless other cruel teenagers had once called it, and set off.

I felt sick to think that he was travelling for the first time without Mark or me, and though he had his 'toy of the moment' for company, I worried that he may become distressed or confused and the escort who sat with the children would be unable to calm him. Every scenario ran through my head, except, of course, the reality. Harry apparently sat quite happily on the bus as it collected children on the route to the school and its staff who were waiting to greet him with the enthusiasm and joy of long lost friends.

I was sad for Harry to be leaving not only the Children's Centre and the staff who had grown to love him, but also Oliver. For the first time, my boys were separated during the daytime. Although Harry rarely interacted with Oliver, the staff told me that Oliver was clearly missing his brother's presence. Because of this, and for reasons of logistical convenience, the transport from school dropped Harry back at the Centre each evening, even though he was unimpressed by Oliver's clear joy in seeing him again.

In no time at all we were in a new routine which soon became a familiar arrangement, and for a while, life returned to our sleep-deprived, laughter-filled guessing game version of normality.

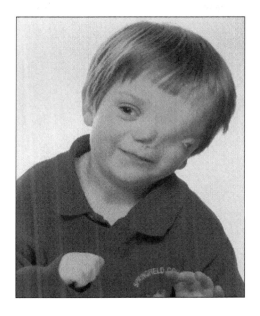

Harry the Musician and Oliver the Comedian

I was enjoying my teaching training, but it was intense. As ever, I invested everything I had in terms of energy into being successful. It is hard enough for anyone who is simultaneously juggling a family and studying, but I had one other factor which added pressure to my situation.

Harry didn't care much for sleeping and existed on only a few hours. Every night was eventful, every day a tiring battle with myself to stay focused and alert. The consultant had prescribed melatonin, a hormone that is produced by the pineal gland in the brain, to regulate Harry's body clock, but it increased his hyperactivity – Tigger became the Tasmanian Devil for a while. We stopped it pretty quickly.

As a barber, Mark worked incredibly hard, and as his busiest day was Saturday, he took Wednesdays off work instead. I never complained about this as I knew it would be the case when we decided to start a family, but it meant he had Wednesdays without his family and we had Saturdays without him. At times it felt lonely for me, and I'm sure it did for him, too. When we thought about the quality time that we spent together, it totalled four days a month – just Sundays. This made me sad.

To combat our blues, we tried to enjoy the Sundays that we had together then make the most of the time to ourselves. Mark hardly went out, but had a couple of holidays abroad with friends. I, on the other hand, couldn't face the thought of leaving the boys for that long and chose instead to socialise with my girlfriends on nights out. Mark and I rarely went out together as Harry's bedtime routine was so unpredictable. He was challenging for us to manage, let alone for family members who supported us. And so we coped with the life we shared quite differently with less consideration for each other and more concern for the moments of 'freedom' from being Mum or Dad.

That's not to say that we didn't enjoy being parents. Any mum or dad will know that you can be at your wits' end with a child for a whole host of reasons, and then one little moment, or look, or touch can melt you and it's all forgotten again. Our boys were no different.

Oliver was such a cheeky boy and would do anything to make us laugh. He would wear my nan's hat and scarf and mimic her for us, encouraged by our laughter and pleasure. The programmes that he watched on TV were brought to life by him in our home – I have video footage, which will be shown when he turns 18, of his killer dance moves while he sang the theme tune to *LazyTown* as the health-obsessed Icelandic superhero, Sportacus. When the production came to a local theatre, Oliver was there in full costume, complete with a delicate moustache courtesy of my kohl eyeliner pencil. His chatting was incessant, and every now and then I would hear a word that was far beyond the vocabulary of a three-year-old. I marvelled at him and his ever-receptive mind and knowledge-hungry soul.

Harry, although less able to communicate, was still able to amuse us and show that he had emotions other than frustration. He would clamber onto our knees and sit facing us, grab both hands and lurch forwards and backwards until we sang *Row, Row, Row the Boat* so that he could join in with sounds and the odd words that he knew. He would pre-empt a warning from us as he dared to do something forbidden, such as climbing to help himself to biscuits, and slowly creep towards his target with a shady glance over his shoulder, his cheeky smile clearly saying, "I know I shouldn't be doing this."

One talent that he never struggled with was playing on the keyboard. With his love of all things noisy and flashy, it was natural for us to buy him a children's keyboard, and for a while we used to think he had hit the 'demo' key and was aimlessly playing along. How wrong we were. Harry knew, although he couldn't always sing them, a few nursery rhymes by now, and in no time he was playing them on his keyboard. His fingers didn't hesitate over the keys, but flew across them as he instinctively knew where the tune should take them next.

When we acquired a second-hand piano, I took dozens of videos of Harry happily playing various nursery rhymes and, over time, general songs or tunes that he'd heard on the television or from toys. He taught himself to play as effortlessly and efficiently as he had taught himself colours, shapes and numbers from his many phonics boards. Predicable, safe technology could teach him where unpredictable and spontaneous humans failed. I felt saddened and relieved in equal measure that he was interacting in a way that was helping him, even if it wasn't with the people around him.

Although he was still receiving speech and language therapy at school and home, his progress was slow and inconsistent. He would make more sounds at home than he would at nursery, which made assessment difficult and predictions for his development almost impossible. In addition to this, we were fluent in 'Harry', interpreting the grunts, signals and sounds that he made. Sometimes we forgot just how hard it was for new people in Harry's life to understand him.

He still became incredibly frustrated, though, even with us. On more than one occasion, as I sat him on my knee, trying to pacify and distract him, he would throw himself back forcibly and suddenly, splitting my bottom lip as he had done at the aquarium. I would yelp and he would jump from my knee, happy not to be mithered by me, and wander away, sometimes laughing, leaving me bleeding and deflated.

The Triad of Impairment

Taking all of Harry's habits and his developmental progress into account, his speech and language therapist suggested that we have him assessed for autism. It sounds ridiculous to say that this surprised me. I am a sensible and realistic woman, and looking back, it made perfect sense, but at first I was stunned. This was just Harry. He had his quirks and his obsessions, and yes he was developmentally delayed, but it was how he was. It took me a few days to consider the fact that my son might be unfortunate enough to have two conditions to deal with.

We took him for the assessment in February after Mr Mellor, the clinical psychologist, had visited the school a few times to observe Harry and talk with the staff. Mr Mellor explained that in order for Harry to receive a diagnosis of Autistic Spectrum Disorder, he should show significant difficulties in three areas of development or behaviour known as the Triad of Impairment. I remembered this from my psychology degree when I researched with great fascination the background of ASD and ways in which it manifested itself, and it felt strange to be revisiting the topic in the context of my own life.

I did smile briefly inside at the mention of the Triad of Impairment which sounded like somewhere that Spock and Captain Kirk might have visited on the Starship Enterprise. Actually, it's not a bad analogy to compare a child's world of autism with uncharted territory.

We were asked about Harry's communication skills. While he had begun to chatter to himself at times, it was a mixture of unrecognisable babble and word approximations. "Iss ay" would mean "This way" and "Ox off" would mean "Socks off". Although he was trying hard to communicate with us, he generally preferred to copy whatever we said to him, like an echo.

"Good morning, Harry."

"U orning, Ayyee."

"Do you want some toast?"

"'Oast."

"And a drink?"

"Dyink."

He wouldn't nod or shake his head to show yes or no. Occasionally he used a few gestures, like waving when I asked him to say goodbye or lifting his arms to be picked up, but generally he was still hand leading (anyone at all) to wherever or whatever he wanted.

Mr Mellor had observed that Harry's contextual understanding had improved slightly and he could make a choice between two common object picture cards, shapes and numbers. I explained that although he seemed to respond to the intonation of voice as much as the meaning of the words, he never made eye contact with the people around him. It was possible to guess Harry's mood from the amount of rocking, jumping or arm flapping he did and the noises that he made, but he never attempted to share his feelings with anyone. I watched him experience his world as if he were behind glass, unconcerned whether I was there or not.

Mr Mellor summarised Harry's difficulties in communication as delayed speech and language skills, limited evidence of purposeful communication, evidence of echolalia, limited use of gestures and limited evidence of imaginative play. Harry had one of the three pieces of a jigsaw I hoped we wouldn't complete.

Next up was Social Development and Play. From watching Harry at school and talking to the staff, Mr Mellor told us what we already knew about our boy and his 'friends'. He tolerated children unless they tried to touch his toys – woe betide the child who wanted to play with a toy that Harry was using. He could not share with them.

His fascination with crying children had continued from the first occasion at nursery. He would stand close to watch a wailing child with his head tilted and body still. Then he would jump up and down and laugh. The louder the child cried, the harder Harry laughed. I only ever found it amusing as I knew that he wasn't being cruel, but Oliver never saw the funny side when his tears were the source of Harry's entertainment, so I had to learn to keep my giggles in check when Harry was (often!) inappropriate.

Other than these moments, Harry preferred his own company and played alone. Even the word 'alone' feels bleak to me, and I used to feel so sad that Harry could be alone in a roomful of people, although at times, I was beginning to feel the same way.

As at home, he dragged school staff by the hand to wherever he needed them to be in order for him to obtain what he wanted, and showed little preference for which adult he approached. At home, he was observed interacting better with me, Mark and my nan, who adored him more every day. She loved her grandsons and called them "My boys". He was still choosing cause and effect toys both at home and school and wasn't showing any signs of imaginative play, although Mr Mellor was astonished when I showed him a video of Harry playing the piano. He had questioned my definition of 'playing' and asked whether I meant that Harry enjoyed hitting the keys. I felt great pride as he watched my little Beethoven's fingers skimming the piano keys like flat rocks across a still pool, with patience, passion and precision. This was definitely not 'hitting the keys', and I was thrilled that Harry's talents, as well as his difficulties, were acknowledged as part of the assessment.

His difficulties in social interaction were listed as: variable eye contact; not being at the level of sharing or showing or offering comfort; does not play interactively with other children; contact with adults merely as a way of getting something; decreased range of facial expressions. There was no evidence that Harry wanted to share his interest or excitement of things with others.

Piece two in the bag. One part of the Triad of Impairment to go.

The final part of the assessment focused on Rigid, Repetitive and Obsessive Behaviour and Sensory Interests. I believed that this aspect would be less significant for Harry. Although he liked to know his routine for the day, he wasn't unduly upset by any changes (other than the car reversing – that sent him into meltdown, and I don't *think* it was just because of my driving). He wasn't attached to one or two specific objects, but he did have a strong interest in Peppa Pig and enjoyed watching it repeatedly – we did not share his love of the Pig family – and he did favour specific toys from time to time. He would regularly line them up precisely, a collection of ducks, bears, phonics board, vehicles arranged in such a way that he knew if any of them were moved so much as an inch. This sentenced them to remain like that until he decided otherwise. This behaviour was certainly rigid, but I wasn't convinced that it qualified as obsessive.

However, his senses were very acute. He became extremely distressed by the sound of the hoover, although I didn't mind this inconvenience, and the hairdryer, which caused more problems as I was not prepared to look like a scarecrow 24/7. Other loud noises, such as food blenders, motorbikes, lawnmowers and hand dryers in public toilets, also upset him greatly and he would smack the side of his head in a fierce rage as he screamed to block them out.

He was greatly affected by textures. While he preferred stodgy 'finger foods', he would scream and throw himself around if a thin string of cheese was hanging down from a piece of pizza and touched his lips before he ate it. That piece of food would be thrown across the room and never forgiven for its violation of Harry's lip. Often I would resemble a dog in the park, retrieving the abandoned pieces of food.

Food that was juicy was another no-no, and anything that needed to be bitten would be launched away too. This limited his diet considerably, and meant that I soon became the master of disguising new foods within familiar ones. What parent doesn't mash vegetables into potatoes, though?

Harry used his body a lot to cope with whatever internal acrobatics he was experiencing. When he became excited, his arms would tense at the side of his body before shaking in small controlled movements, almost as if he were vibrating. He still enjoyed rocking backwards and forwards and jumping for long periods of time on the trampoline, sofas and beds. Often he would bounce on his toes while flapping his arms or tapping his tummy with his hands, and occasionally he would laugh for no apparent reason. No one knew why he did these things, although a course I attended a few years later suggested that this is a strategy that autistic children use to balance their frenetic internal energy, which otherwise would feel far too overwhelming. I quite liked that theory, but Harry could never help me to discover how true it was for him.

In his report, Mr Mellor referenced Harry's 'startling aptitude' for picking up a tune and later playing it on his piano. While I had believed my child to be either the reincarnation of Beethoven or destined for the *Britain's Got Talent* TV show, it turned out that the knowledge that one key would always make the same note meant that Harry learnt to play by association, much like he had done with the letters or numbers of a phonics board. This was merely him demonstrating the power of an autistic mind.

We had our diagnosis – another label to drape around his neck like a luggage tag on Paddington Bear.

My Fault?

I knew that Mr Mellor's diagnosis would change nothing about Harry, and I hoped that, from a positive perspective, he may be entitled to more support. But I felt like I had failed him again.

As scary as the unknown is, Harry's development prior to the diagnosis of autism gave me hope that he would find his own way through whatever was holding him back. Once the psychologist confirmed him to be on the Autistic Spectrum, though, I knew that he was wandering within the labyrinth of his alternatively wired brain. Would my Theseus ever be able to find his way out?

As Mr Mellor explained how Harry met the criteria to receive the diagnosis, we nodded in calm acceptance, but my mind was racing. What about Oliver – was his brother lost to him now? How could I explain that Harry wasn't consciously choosing to push him away or ignore him when Oliver, deflated and lonely, asked why Harry wouldn't play with him. Mr Mellor recommended some books that I could read to Oliver to try to explain, but he was far too young to be having to consider topics such as autism.

The kayak on which I was, ever more confidently, navigating our uncertain rivers capsized again and I was left gasping for breath while smiling confidently at the psychologist. My poor boys – separated by another glass divide. I felt cheated on their behalf.

Again I felt guilty. I was still battling, although nowhere near as much as I had during the first couple of years, with the demons within me that heaped blame into my soul like coals onto a fire that I was fighting hard not to be consumed by. All of the professionals had told me emphatically that Goldenhar syndrome was not the result of anything that I had or had not done, but having researched autism, I knew that some medical studies pointed in the direction of genetics when theorising about its origins. My cousin on my father's side is autistic, and I pictured a rogue gene swimming through my veins until it chose Harry as its recipient. My body. My genes. My fault.

We left the assessment and I sat in the car, sobbing into my hands – the sort of crying that shakes your shoulders and makes your throat ache. Mark had driven to the assessment in his own car, so by the time we met up again at home, I had composed myself enough to talk about the positive outcomes from the meeting and the next steps we needed to take. We never discussed with each other how we felt about the diagnosis, didn't take the time to swear and cry and laugh and relax together. We just continued with our lives and made the most of the latest news. In fact, I don't recall getting upset many more times after that at all, choosing instead to distract myself with the boys and my job.

We informed Springfield of Harry's diagnosis. As a school which already supported children on the Autistic

Spectrum, it didn't need to make any significant changes to his daily routine and life there – one of the many reasons why I am glad we never pushed for a mainstream school place for him.

His teacher, Lisa, loved him. I remember during one of the many meetings that I had with her about his progress, she laughed as she explained a learning activity that the children did in which they completed something at a three-sided workstation before moving on to the next. Harry started with just a few workstations, but was soon working on several, each of which got him closer to the treat at the end. However, unlike many of the children who applied their 'rigid thinking' to following the rules, Harry would walk to the box at the end of the workstations, take the sweet treat and then complete the activities while enjoying his reward. He was hilarious and had no idea just how entertaining he was – my cheeky superstar and Lisa's lovable 'rat bag'.

Lisa and her team worked hard to support Harry's learning, and were always sharing their successes with us so that we could try them at home to reinforce the message. I was full of admiration for the staff who worked with Harry – for their ideas and constant re-evaluation and evolving plans. His love of noisy toys was curbed, and they were restricted to being rewards only once he had completed his learning. He was beginning to use a 'now and next' board to sequence his day and was definitely making sounds which were meaningful to him rather than pointless babble. Although we couldn't always understand what he was saying, he was slowly becoming more patient with us as we tried.

Harry Houdini

We were all making steady progress together and our version of life even began to feel easy. However, there were occasional harsh reality checks that would pluck me from complacency and drop me onto my toes again.

One such day was a warm, sunny Saturday afternoon in August 2009. Nan and I were busy cleaning up and tidying the toys which had been strewn around the house by Harry. Oliver was playing in the garden, and I knew exactly where he was as I could follow the loud and surprisingly deep tones as he chatted away to himself.

Harry was entertaining himself in the lounge, lining up toys and pressing sound effect buttons. But then there was quiet. Now in most family households, peace and quiet almost always means that there is some mischief going on, but in my house, silence panics me like the siren of a wailing fire alarm.

Harry had gone. I don't know how I knew it, but I knew.

I flew through the rooms upstairs, hoping to see him bouncing on a bed or with his head stuck in a toy chest while his arms rotated backwards cartoon style, scattering toys behind him. From there, I dashed downstairs and repeated the search from room to room, knowing the entire time that it was futile. I yelled for Nan, asked if Harry was with her. She heard the panic in my voice and I heard it in her reply.

Outside, Oliver had stopped playing and was watching me like a statue, frozen and stunned by the sudden chaos. The side gate was open ever so slightly. Not only had Harry managed to get through the string that we had wrapped around the gate to secure it, but he had closed it behind him to cover his tracks.

I shouted that I was going to find him and ran, faster than I have ever run, leaving Oliver with Nan. Once at the edge of the drive, I had no way of knowing which way to turn. The house was in a quiet semi-rural area and we were surrounded by fields and dirt tracks. He could have been anywhere.

I ran left, my bare feet oblivious to the rough stones I was stamping across. All manner of sinister thoughts crossed my mind – what if Harry had been taken, the gate closed to give the perpetrator extra valuable minutes to put distance between us? What if Harry had fallen somewhere, unable to call for me? The terror of Harry's Spanish Houdini episode returned to haunt me as I ran, screaming his name in the hope that he was still close enough to hear me.

A small crossroads lay before me. To my left and right, roads headed towards more fields and town respectively. Before me, a dirt path narrowed as it dipped out of sight. A red sports car turned right past me as I stood paralysed in the middle of the road.

I put out my hand and shouted, "Have you seen a little boy?"

The male driver replied with a sentence that terrified me to my core. I wanted to pass out with fear.

"I've just seen a bloke carrying a child further up there." He motioned to the road he was just leaving, to my left.

I fled back to the house, grabbed my car keys and phone. Still bare-footed, I sped out of the drive to search for my boy. I drove to the top of the road on which the man said he had seen the boy, sobbing and begging out loud, "Please don't be Harry. Please don't be Harry," but at the same time desperately wanting to find him.

There was no sign of anyone anywhere, which wasn't unusual in the sleepy village, but I felt alone in the world with no idea what to do. Driving back down the road, I skidded to a halt at the crossroads and rang Mark. By this time, some of the neighbours had come out of their houses, wondering who was screaming and why. As Mark answered the phone, I was telling them all that Harry was missing and I couldn't find him anywhere.

"What?" Mark's voice jumped through the phone receiver. He was driving through the town as I called him and was passing a police car, so he told them what was happening. Within minutes I heard the sirens approaching, and a mixture of relief and terror made me gag on my own emotion.

Officers in two cars went straight to the brook which trickled behind the cottages while another car approached me to ask what Harry was wearing.

"I don't know," I said, hysterical by now, "but he's very distinctive. He's only got one eye and he can't talk. He can't shout for me if he needs me!"

Soon I wasn't even talking anymore, but making an ear-piercing wailing noise. Every part of my body was shaking.

The neighbours had scattered and I could hear various voices shouting Harry's name, out of sight around me. I jumped back into my car and turned it around to face the crossroads again. I had searched left, the police had headed right, and so I drove forwards down the dirt path. As the road dipped down it began to narrow and I could get no further. Slowly I reversed backwards, checking in the mirror as I weaved my way past a row of cars to my left.

As I saw the junction again, I turned to face the dirt track. Through the overgrown hedgerows and bushes, I saw a flash of turquoise. Getting out, I walked to the front of my car on legs shaking so fiercely that I thought they would give way and watched in slow motion as that dot of turquoise got bigger. Then, through a gap in the bushes, I saw Harry.

Slowly, without a care in the world, he came bouncing up the small path, clutching a phonics board in his hand and humming a tune.

"He's HERE!" I screamed. Just as he got close enough for me to grab him, my legs gave way.

My wonderful neighbour Betty was at my side in a flash and caught me as she simultaneously scooped Harry towards us both. We sat in a heap on the floor, my arms around him as I sobbed into his hair and Betty with her arms around us both, until Mark and the police arrived. I was convinced that I was going to be sick, but once I was back in the house and had stopped violently shuddering, I felt only exhaustion. Every part of my body ached from tension. It had been only about 30 minutes since I had realised Harry had left, and yet I felt sure I had aged another 10 years.

Oliver's Trauma

Oliver was distraught. Looking at that day through his eyes, I realise he had been happily playing in the garden only to have his tranquillity destroyed by my shouts as I flew past him and ran off, leaving him with my nan. He was already cautious, always wanting to know our whereabouts, but moments like this – which wasn't the last one, but was by far the longest and most dramatic – added to Oliver's growing conviction that I would leave him.

If we were in the lounge and I walked into the kitchen without warning him, I would have to dash back as he wailed in blind panic. Following Harry's monumentally traumatic escapade, I had to inform Oliver where I was going every time I left his sight. Often he would come with me, even if that meant tearing himself away from his beloved TV programmes or songs. Room to room he accompanied me like a shadow, and on the rare occasion that I was able to go for a shower and leave him downstairs, I knew it wouldn't be long before he was standing in the hall, yelling my name. He would ask four or five times per morning what his daily routine would be and who would be collecting him from the after school club he attended at the Children's Centre, and he started to have nightmares about being locked in a car which was rolling away from us. I didn't know what to do to help him, other than constantly reassure him that I wouldn't leave.

Although it sounds obvious to connect the activity around Harry absconding and Oliver's anxiety, I didn't consider the significance of it for quite some time, so while we tried hard to ensure that Oliver knew where we were all of the time, Mark and I were both incredibly frustrated. Not only did we have to keep a watchful eye on Harry day and night, constantly assessing any risks, but we also had to announce our movements like a satellite navigation system for Oliver. At times, I felt like I was going mad. Plus I was tired.

I had completed my teacher training and was waiting to start my first year as a qualified teacher. This and raising the boys felt like my greatest achievements and I was incredibly proud, but every joyful moment was overshadowed by sleep deprivation and an increasing loneliness. Maybe I was post-natally depressed. I had never given myself time to explore that theory before, pushing it to one side and creating an action plan of how to move forward at lightning pace. I don't know for sure, but I was feeling lost, the type of sadness that I had experienced just after the boys' birth. It smothered me like a blanket and stifled my every moment. I was crying. A lot. And I wasn't sharing any of it with Mark.

He was working, busy improving the 'forever home' we had pushed our budget to buy, and I was voluntarily drowning in paperwork and laughing only with my friends at work or on nights out. Home was a grey zone

– not the oasis of calm into which we could all collapse at the end of a hectic day. We talked about our days and relayed information about the boys to each other. There were no arguments, but maybe that was part of the problem as the wider, significant issues beyond the boys were left unaddressed between us. Family issues that tested his loyalty and my patience. Slowly, the things we didn't say or do chipped away at my confidence about us as a couple. Over time and without us realising it, our relationship disintegrated.

A Sad Decision

In the September of 2009 I told Mark that I was unhappy with the way things were between us. I had plenty of friends and I didn't need another; I needed a husband. Unfortunately, by the time I mentioned it, I knew that we were beyond repair.

We agreed to try counselling, but in all honestly, we went with different agendas – Mark to convince me to stay; me to convince him to let me go. It was never going to help us.

Making the decision to leave Mark was the hardest and the easiest decision I have ever made. Hard, because he is a good man, and remains to this day my friend. We hadn't long been married; we'd made promises to each other in front of our family and friends, which I had truly believed we would keep. I had loved him and we had shared some incredible moments together which I still treasure. Hurting him was the last thing I wanted to do.

I was also well aware that my selfish decision would destroy my family. My boys would migrate from the statistically safe and secure category of 'raised by both parents' to the uncertain and grim predictions for the future of children 'from a divorced background'. I knew this and considered it long and hard before I talked to Mark. Again, a fatal error – I should have allowed him to hear my thought process, like Oliver needed to hear descriptions of my movements and whereabouts, and given him the chance to work through it all with me. Though I am not sure it would have changed the outcome.

It was an easy decision because I was becoming someone I no longer recognised. I was sad all the time, and any enjoyment I had took effort. Much of my laughter was forced.

One evening, cooking dinner at home, I was gripped by a pain that I can only imagine felt like a heart attack. A sharp stabbing constriction snatched my breath away and knocked me literally off my feet. As I slid to the floor with my back to the cupboards, an involuntary sob escaped my throat and I felt physically empty. Hollow and lost. I have never felt so alone as I did in that moment.

Oliver walked into the kitchen and saw me huddled in the corner like a pile of discarded dirty clothes. He stood above me and wrapped his little arms over my crumpled body and shushed my tears as I had done many times for him. Years earlier, I had done the very same thing for my own mother after my father had told her that he was taking my brother and me away from her.

In that moment, I knew that I couldn't carry on living like this. My son couldn't be my saviour each time I crumbled, having to grow up with the responsibility of being my protector and guard. To be the mother my boys deserved, I needed to be mentally well enough to face the challenges that lay ahead for all of us. I also needed

Oliver to know that I was strong enough to live without him as my emotional crutch, freeing him up to explore the infinite possibilities that lay before him in a world that I hoped he would discover. He was very much like me and I knew that he would stay at my side, faithful and loyal, for as long as he thought I needed him. That couldn't happen, and so my decision to leave was made.

Night Time Antics

Mark helped me to find a place close to our house that I could rent. Once I had signed the lease, I took the boys to see it.

As we pulled up on the drive, Oliver held my hand and said, "We're going to live here, aren't we, Mummy?" The wise and wonderful soul of my intuitive and sensitive boy knew what I was about to tell him even before I could begin.

I moved out at the end of October 2009, taking some plates and cutlery with me and a credit card to start a new life on a shoestring budget and a diet of determination and optimism. I had bought beds and wardrobes for us all, as well as a cheap and cheerful sofa. Most of the other items I had were donated by my incredible friends and family, and my nan was the charity shop champion at finding all sorts of bargains. My small semi-detached home with no real garden to speak of was a far cry from the beautiful, detached family home and luscious green lawns that I was leaving, but as I moved the bits that I had in, I made it a home for me and the boys.

They adapted incredibly well after the move. Although Harry was unnerved by his new surroundings for a while, he soon settled and adjusted to a new routine of 'girl night' and 'boy night'. Oliver asked the question every morning and I always made sure that I told both him and Harry whether they would be with me or their dad that evening. I believe that Harry knew more than he could express, and including him in those conversations was vital to how well he coped with such big changes.

Although we lived separately, Mark and I continued to do things together with the boys for a while. Part of me wondered whether I needed some space from him to give me the opportunity to miss him as my husband, but as time passed I realised just how much I valued him only as a friend. While that sounds harsh, the lives of our boys have been enriched by having parents who get along rather than the toxic situation that was ruining their mother. I am incredibly proud of the parenting team Mark and I are.

*****

Slowly, I started to see a change in myself. I don't think it is any coincidence that this correlated with the sleep I was now getting on the nights that the boys slept at their dad's. Anyone who thinks that sleep deprivation is a tired man's excuse for poor functioning has obviously never experienced it. It is renowned for being used as an effective technique when interrogating prisoners, and research consistently provides evidence that prolonged sleep deprivation affects pupils' attainment at school and employees' performance at work.

It's more than just being tired. It's the sort of tired that slows your brain and alters your mood, delays your reactions and dulls your responses. It's like a fog that clings to your clothes and follows you everywhere, diluting each of your senses as you drag your body through each day, under pressure to think and perform 100% efficiently. The antithesis of rational logic and emotion.

Whereas I had previously functioned on around four or five hours of broken sleep every night, I was now sleeping deeply and solidly for three nights a week. My battered brain and sluggish body were receiving the energy transfusion to regenerate that they had been deprived of. I hadn't realised just how much of an effort it had been for me to be a full-time teacher, housewife and mum. Yes, I know there are millions of women who juggle these commitments happily, but I couldn't. I was exhausted and fighting self-loathing and guilt that, every now and then, raised their heads to ensure they weren't forgotten before submerging below my consciousness again. I had been battling with myself, and I didn't even realise it until much later.

As time passed, my mental health improved, but my physical health was still playing catch up. Yes, I felt better for resting, but my teaching workload was increasing and Harry was still an insomniac version of Tigger. I would put Oliver to bed while Harry bounced, squealed and flapped downstairs, and then I would sit with him while we both listened to the soothing, melodic classical tunes of Baby TV and watched the lava lamp-style blobs merge and separate on the screen. Just like life at the old house, he would finally fall asleep next to me at around 11pm and I would edge away so that I could mark books, plan lessons and prepare resources. Moving him often disturbed him, and so I waited until he was in a deep sleep before I dared attempt it.

I would often work until 1am after putting Harry to bed, but by 3am he would be awake again and fully refreshed for the day ahead, unlike me. If he didn't want to be the conductor of all things musical and flashing, then he would clap and squeal in delight while bouncing on the furniture, or climb up on the worktops, scavenging for biscuits like a child who had never been fed. He got a great amount of pleasure from opening the oven and testing the spring hinges of its door by bouncing on it like a DIY trampoline. Nothing and nowhere was safe, and so if Harry was up, so was I.

I would lie on the sofa and watch him play, often dragging him to me in the hope that a warm cuddle would soothe him back to sleep for an hour. Instead, he would bury me in the toys he adored, in particular a highly annoying ball popper that fired plastic balls into the air, synchronised with a harsh and irritating tune. Alternatively, he would take my hand and bend the fingers right back before stroking the smooth, taut skin in captivated fascination until I squealed and wriggled free. Harry loved a reaction and so that game was one of his favourites. It wasn't one of mine. But that little face, the one big, beautiful eye and cheeky smile, would melt me every time. That is one of his gifts, and so it is very hard to be angry with Harry for long.

He was still fighting to express himself with the few words he had. Although the symbols that I had brought with me to the new house worked for some items, his understanding and knowledge of words seemed to be improving more than his ability to covey them, so the unspoken words paced the cage of his brain like a hungry lion. Frustrated, he would slap his head repeatedly and cry out or throw himself to the floor in temper, writhing and screaming. I could see and feel his frustration, but I was helpless to do anything other than try to calm him and guess at his message. It was like playing charades without any clues.

Fleecy Green Blanket

For a long time, my mum had suggested an alternative approach to helping Harry: craniosacral therapy. I hadn't heard of it and I was reluctant to look into it, partly because I didn't have the money to pay for private treatments, and partly because I felt that to ask for support was yet another sign that I had failed as a mother. Mum brought leaflets which I left unread and gave me a telephone number which remained un-dialled.

However, sometime at the beginning of 2010, I read a true-life account of parents with an autistic son who were struggling to help him while falling apart as a family. I identified with a lot of the things they wrote about, and when they talked of craniosacral therapy and the immense benefit that it had had on the entire family unit, my interest was aroused and I agreed to take Harry for a session. Mark was sceptical, but agreed that we needed to try something to help Harry navigate his way through a life which was tormenting and torturing him.

Our first appointment with Nicola was on 12 March 2010 when my boys were four years old. Initially I just took Harry. Nicola works on an energetic as well as a practical level, and knowing what I know now about Harry, tampering with his frequency was always going to be a challenge.

We made our introductions and I explained the history of my boys' birth, how we had come to this point and what I hoped to achieve from the sessions. As we chatted, Harry paced around the room, touching anything he could get his hands on. Nicola described him in the notes she has kindly given to me as *active, unsettled and determined* – a polite way of saying the Tasmanian Devil on a mission. I sat on the floor with my back against the door as he tried more than once to get out and thrashed around, violently objecting to the session.

A violin which is well strung but not tuned may be happy with its strings just as they are. Harry was that violin. Nicola was tuning him energetically, against his will and understanding, and I think now that he was simply scared.

Nicola played some relaxing music and Harry calmed enough to sit with me beneath a fleecy green blanket and allow her to work with us both. It was draining and I wasn't sure what that first session achieved – he was even more hyper than usual for the week that followed. His sleep was worse and he appeared supercharged, but the energy injection from the session hadn't affected me in the same way. What already felt like a battle became even more exhausting.

Mark suggested we leave the therapy there. It clearly wasn't helping Harry, and had in fact only made things tougher. At this point, I need to digress slightly to tell you something which will explain my decision to ignore Harry's dad's wishes.

My grandad had been a spiritual medium and my nan a healer. I spent much of my childhood in spiritualist services, which I thoroughly enjoyed, so maybe I grew up a little bit more in tune with my higher self and energy than most people.

One night in September 2001, I was passing my grandparents' house quite late in the evening and had the urge to call in. I had the usual internal dialogue to debate the idea, but the urge to pop in was too strong to ignore.

Grandad had been a long-distance lorry driver in his day. Knowing that Mark and I were driving to Scotland the next day, he cupped my face in his hands as I left, wished me a great journey, and said, "I'll be with you all the way."

I shouted, "Love you both," as I closed the door.

Grandad died just 15 minutes after I left their home. If I hadn't listened to the voice that urged me to go in, I would never have had that moment, one which I still treasure to this day. From there I promised always to listen to the voice. The voice even has an identity for me. She is Flo, and in times of struggle, doubt, sadness or confusion, I try to hear her and let her guide me.

After Harry's intense first session with Nicola, no one would have blamed me for leaving it there, but Flo said to persevere. So, guided by this, I told Mark that I wanted to give it six sessions and then decide. Just five more weeks and then we would do whatever was needed.

Not only did we continue to have those sessions, but now, almost seven years later, we still go and see Nicola, and she has helped us in ways I can't begin to explain. Reading through Nicola's notes, I clearly see the progress that Harry made during the first few months. Although he was initially distressed and fought her efforts to help, he became calmer, more familiar with the routine of visiting and more accepting of the therapy she offered. His head-banging lessened as his patience improved, and he was trying to use more of the words that were trapped in his mind. It was as if the therapy was channelling all that he already had but was not equipped to express effectively.

After six weeks, his school commented on a marked improvement in his language development, and he was enjoying the sessions – even though they were still incredibly intense and draining for us all.

This isn't to say Harry was transformed. He was still temperamental. He was hitting Oliver and biting children at school. His sleep was an issue, and although he was going to bed at 10pm, he was awake from 1am. I was constantly trying to think of solutions.

In one of the early sessions, I told Nicola that I had to work really hard sometimes to be patient with Harry through the exhaustion, frustration and daily battles. This may sound harsh, but it's a reality of a life we never chose. Some days were harder than others; some challenges seemed never-ending. It's not to say that I didn't love Harry for the funny, highly intelligent, mischievous cuddle monster that he was, but some days were bloody tough.

An unexpected by-product of taking Harry to the sessions was the space I had to offload – to be honest about how lost I was feeling and how exhausted I was, physically, emotionally and mentally. I didn't do this lightly as I rarely shared the extent of my feelings with anyone other than my mum. It felt like a sign of weakness to say that I wasn't coping, and so many people were telling me what a great job I was doing and how inspiring I was that I felt I had to live up to their perception of who I was. Crumbling and complaining was not an option, but behind the smile, I was imploding. The toxic thoughts I had about my own abilities as a mum were corroding my self-esteem.

On more than one occasion, Nicola wrote in her notes *I think it was Charlene who needed today's session.* I do believe that I always had it in me to be the mum my boys deserve, but Nicola ironed me out, topped me up and calmed my fractious inner self so that I could come from a place of energetic strength and grounding. She has no idea how grateful I am to her for that.

Oliver also began to have sessions with Nicola. Reading the notes from those sessions has been tough. My chatty, friendly, inquisitive, comedian boy wished that he could break his arm to have time with me at home, and wasn't sure that he wanted to be alive some days because life with a brother who hit him and never told him that he loved him made him so sad. To know this physically hurts me, but if by sharing it, I help one parent recognise that they are not the only one who is battling, and that the siblings will struggle in many ways more than the unique child ever will, then it will be worth it.

Oliver was lost and angry, but he had a safe space to talk through those issues with Nicola. The therapy sessions we had together not only helped him get his thoughts out, but gave us time to cuddle together under the fleecy green blanket. It was Oliver's request that all three of us had a session together, so at times we were a trio, and at other times it was one of the boys and me alone. Oliver now is fantastic at talking through his emotions, and although he still struggles with his self-esteem at times, and separation anxiety stops him enjoying things like school trips, he has grown up knowing that therapy is good. Talking is good. Asking and finding help when you struggle is good. I hope he continues to value this as he grows.

Without doubt we all, both individually and as a family, benefitted and continue to benefit from Nicola's expertise, support and the time just to stop and focus on ourselves. Well done, Flo.

The Greatest Thing I Ever Did

Oliver's constant running commentary and questions used to drive me insane when he was young (now, in addition he sings constantly and talks through his sleep), but I have never chastised or stopped him. I always wanted him to know that he could talk, even if it was at me more often than with me.

One evening, as we sat on his bed putting his pyjamas on after a bath, he hit me with a question that makes my heart sink to this day.

"Mummy?"

"Yes, Oliver."

"Why do you always say Harry is special but you don't say I am special?"

I was stunned. In my attempt to explain to Oliver why his brother looked so different, hit him instead of played with him, ignored him instead of chatted with him and always attracted a crowd of unwanted spectators, I had said that it was because Harry was special. Of course, I had meant 'different', 'disabled', 'autistic', but it had felt cruel to say these things and so I had used 'special' as an umbrella term. I had never, for a moment, considered that Oliver would hear special in the way that every other child would hear it.

Faced with the wide-eyed sadness of my four-year-old son, I felt like I had failed him beyond words. So, explaining my incredible error, I cuddled and kissed my older son (Oliver will tell you that those three minutes really do count) and apologised. I said I was so sorry that he had felt like that, and when I said special, I meant that Harry was different. A bit lost in his own world.

Around the same time, Oliver kept asking why God had sent Harry to us. Why us specifically? Why couldn't he have gone to another family instead who would have looked after him?

I said that when God was looking for a mummy for Harry, He knew that the mummy would feel really sad sometimes, and so He would have to send another baby who would make her smile. I told Oliver that Harry came to us because God knew that we would look after him, but Oliver came to me as my gift. I told him that I loved him more than the moon and the stars and that he filled a place in my heart that could burst because I was so proud he was mine. I told him that on the days when I felt I was a rubbish mummy because Harry was having a tantrum or not sleeping or generally being hard work, I looked at him – Oliver – and knew I was doing a good job because he was amazing. I told him that of all the wonderful things I had ever done, *he* was the greatest thing.

He seemed happy with these answers, and again I was so thankful that we had been seeing Nicola as I'm not sure he would have asked otherwise.

For a while, I would ask him every day, "What are you?"

He would reply, "The greatest thing you ever did," and I would smother him in kisses until he giggled and pushed me away.

He is almost 12 as I write this now and I still ask him, even now and then, "What are you?"

Sometimes he rolls his eyes and huffs; sometimes he tries to be clever with "Hungry" or "A boy", but we always arrive back at "The greatest thing you ever did" and a hug. And that truth is purer than anything else I will ever know. It is true for both of my boys, without doubt, but that conversation with my four-year-old meant that it will always be the 'special' truth for Oliver.

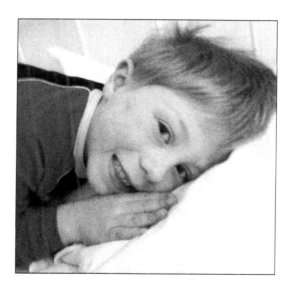

Good Job

My boys were settling well into the routine of girl night and boy night, and we were all getting into the swing of our new arrangements. It was lovely to be able to concentrate on other things besides change. Teaching was going well for me and I loved the rewards of being with the children, although I was still juggling the demands of being an enthusiastic, energised class teacher and an exhausted Harry tamer.

The boys were also settling well into school. Harry's class teacher, Lisa, adored him, but was super firm which he responded well to. She had high expectations of him and knew what he was capable of. Where he was able to convince others (even me at times) that he couldn't do something, Lisa knew it was simply a case of 'wouldn't' and she pushed him. He absolutely loved her, too.

She worked closely in supporting me with the same strategies that he coped well with at school, one being the 'naughty chair' which helped for a while to make him realise the relationship between inappropriate behaviour and a consequence. It worked up until the point where he would sit himself on it and giggle. It was so hard not to laugh with him.

My nan used to say, "He's not as green as he is cabbage looking." It's a hilarious saying that only a woman in her eighties could get away with, but it is true.

Security at school was, as you would expect, tight. Doors had codes on them and high handles that little bodies couldn't reach. This didn't stop Harry Houdini, though. With his one eye, he would watch the code being inputted before pulling a chair up to the door and trying to escape. Often it was to get to toys in other rooms; sometimes it was just for fun.

On one occasion, Lisa raced around looking for him and searched every room. As panic finally set in, she heard the click of a familiar door and went to investigate. Harry was in the head teacher's office, had opened a tall cupboard and was standing on the inside where he could wait unseen until he made his next move.

We all loved the genius mischief maker and his cunning plans. Rather than being angry or concerned, I was thrilled that he could think of such brilliant ideas and had the nerve to try to outsmart the teachers. When he tilts his head and smiles up at you with that one twinkling eye, it's impossible not to melt. Everyone who meets him falls in love with him.

His personality was developing as well as his courage. He was a cake and biscuit fan, and I remember walking into the kitchen one morning to find that Harry had pulled his chair up to the cupboard and was sitting on the worktop with a box of fairy cake mixture.

When I asked what he was doing, he simply shouted, "I yike hake!" which meant I like cake. We baked that day, once I had stopped laughing.

I also remember smiling to myself as I listened to my

boys argue, in Harry's own way, over a toy. The bickering lasted a while before Oliver came running into me.

"Mummy, Harry can talk!"

He was so excited.

It was easy to assume that Harry understood as much as he could express, but I never stopped hoping that one day I would talk to him and he would just reply, in the way that Oliver did, without thinking about it. A reply that I didn't need to structure for him to repeat. A day when I could say, "I love you," and he would say, "I love you, too," without me having to say, "Harry says, love you too, Mummy". I never stopped talking to him, either – not at him, but with him.

One night as we were going to bed, I got his dinosaur teddy and passed it to him.

"Say goodnight to dinosaur, Harry, and put him away."

Harry took the teddy from me, kissed it, put it into the toy chest and said, "Ee oooooooo amorrow." Those moments are like winning the lottery. A second in time when my heart could burst with excitement and happiness; a glimmer of hope for the future and a sign that I'm not *always* talking to myself. I can count on the fingers of both hands the times in Harry's 11 years that he has spontaneously replied, but once you find gold, you keep digging the land.

My clever little monkey. Before long we knew him as Lisa's rat bag and Mummy's superstar. If I said "Harry is Lisa's..." he would shout, "YAT BAG!" He thrived under her care, and to this day, if he does things well, we will all say, "Goooooood jo-ob," in an American drawl, as Lisa did. That's her legacy and we still love her for it now.

After one of his many operations, Lisa made the 100-mile round trip to visit Harry. As he came round from his anaesthetic, the only thing he whispered was, "Gooooood jo-ob". She was so touched.

At home, the mischief continued. The neighbours who shared our drive had grandchildren, and obviously with grandchildren come toys. After randomly bursting into their house and discovering their toy box one day, Harry made it his mission to get around there at any opportunity.

At first, he just dashed out without me realising, so I started to lock the door. Then he worked out how to unlock the door and abscond. Often, I'd hear the deep tones of my neighbour calling, "Charlene!" and laughing as Harry ransacked their toy box.

When I locked the door and removed the key, he was stuck for a while. Until he realised he could leave through the back patio doors and down the side of the house. When Harry has his mind set on something, he's like a guided missile. Thankfully they were lovely neighbours and so it never caused too much stress.

The Habitual Helper

Harry's biggest fan was my nan. Right from the first time she saw the boys, she loved them like they were her own sons. Maybe it was because of our close bond, I don't know, but each and every day she came to see them. She worried when Mark and I moved to our 'forever home' as it was off the beaten track, but she found a bus route. When I moved into the house on my own, it was easier for her to get to us and so she came more often.

She found it hard when the boys went to school, but lived for the weekends when she could sing to them, sit with them, walk with us, make a den and climb inside it with them – not bad for a woman in her mid-eighties. She was a warrior woman and I always hoped to have a fraction of her strength.

At times, though, it was difficult to parent with a sidekick who fed the children chocolate buttons, regardless of the occasion. If a body-thrashing temper tantrum was in full flow, I knew to throw cushions onto the hearth and stand well back until Harry calmed. Nan hated to see him like that and would wade in so that she could force feed him treats – yeah, because more sugar was *exactly* what the moment needed – only to be kicked and scratched.

Harry was also incredibly independent. Despite having only one eye and compromised depth perception, he navigated the stairs without issue. Nan worried and insisted that she held his hand up and down the stairs. I would ask her not to, but she felt I was too harsh and ignored me. Harry pushed her away from him once and she almost toppled down the stairs. Still she persevered, desperate to protect him from any harm at any cost.

It was hard knowing that I was offending her by trying to parent in my own way, but I soon came to realise that it actually wasn't that Nan thought the boys needed her. She needed them. They gave her a sense of purpose. They were like a transfusion of awe, wonder and energy to her veins, and as much as there were times when I wished that she would leave me to my own devices, there are days now when Oliver cries because he misses her, and I'd give anything to watch her force chocolate onto my boys – not that they'd need much forcing!

I realised then that people who are habitual helpers are addicted to the feeling of being needed. It defines them. Who am I to challenge that? And would I be writing this book if it wasn't to serve some need in me to help someone else? Now, I listen to advice, knowing that people are imparting it to help themselves as much as me. Sometimes I follow their advice, sometimes I don't, but I am always grateful for their time. Nan's love taught me that, among many other things.

Nan never understood why I wanted to teach. She saw the impact it had on my hours at home and felt that I should put my own children before a classful of other people's. I saw that, but I knew that I needed to be fulfilled in ways other than as a mother. For me, having my own financial independence and a rewarding job gave me that satisfaction.

But it was getting tougher as Harry's nocturnal adventures continued. In the September of 2010 I was so physically exhausted that I almost passed out at work. My candle was burning fiercely at both ends and I was at breaking point.

I went to the head teacher, who was as understanding of my situation as a boss can be when they are running a school where one person's absence has a knock-on effect. She told me to go home via Harry's school where I was to ask for more help. I found this hard, but I knew I had to do something.

I drove to Harry's school and sat chatting with Lisa. I explained and I cried, and Lisa, as always, gave me some great advice to create a safe and calm area in my tiny box room for Harry to call his own. Then I had some time off work and slept to recharge my batteries like a hibernating hedgehog in the winter.

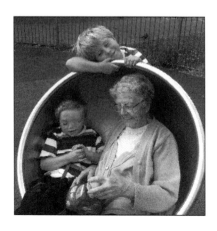

A Little Body at
War with Itself

Towards the end of the year, Harry began to get incredibly grumpy. He returned to his head-banging frustrated behaviours and cried much more than usual. With no way of knowing what was wrong, we all felt helpless and stuck for ideas on what to do.

I visited the doctor to be told that he perhaps had an infection somewhere, and we were given antibiotics to try. Two days later, on 31 December 2010 I came into the kitchen to see Harry's face smeared in fresh bright red blood. Instantly my eyes searched the room for a knife as I was convinced he had cut himself. It was only on closer inspection that I noticed his 'eye' – or rather, the tiny lids that bulged from the side of his head – was bleeding.

I rushed him to A&E. Immediately he was checked into the children's ward and the doctors administered IV fluids and antibiotics while they made a plan. As much as I am not a fan of New Year's Eve, I really hadn't been expecting to spend it on a camp bed in hospital with my little man, but that is where 2011, and a brand new chapter in my life, began.

*****

We spent most of the first week of 2011 in the local hospital, waiting for action and a decision. Harry was grumpy and clearly uncomfortable. I slept at his side, swapping for one night with Mark so that I could see Oliver, and Harry could have some Daddy time. The doctors decided to give Harry an MRI scan to assess the situation and starved him for hours before telling us that they didn't have a space free for him. This happened twice more, and it was clear that the local hospital was just not equipped to deal with such a complex case as Harry.

By 5 January 2011 I had had enough and insisted the doctors call Alder Hey. I knew that the consultants there would have a solution for us, and sure enough, after one call we were transferred to Liverpool. We arrived on 6 January and Harry was admitted to the high dependency unit before being scanned the same day.

On Friday 7 January, he was in theatre having his balloon removed. Just a couple of hours after Harry had gone down to theatre, the surgeon was telling us that the tiny balloon, which had initially given us so much hope for a future for our boy, was infected. He explained that in all his years of surgery, he had never smelt something so bad, and that he had physically gagged on the stench when removing the rotting material from my boy's head.

I wanted to scoop my boy up immediately, kiss his weary head and tell him how sorry I was for not even considering the fact that his body was at war with itself.

The guilt, again, was overwhelming. Little did I know then that I would spend Harry's life thereafter being extra vigilant, mindful that a simple issue could be so much more for the boy who was incapable of telling me.

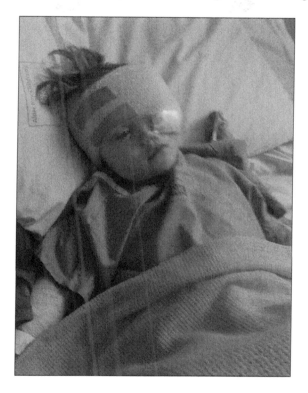

The Wish List

We stayed at Alder Hey for another four days and the change in Harry was remarkable. He was resting and not thrashing around. He was smiling and laughing instead of frowning and distant. He had been in pain and I hadn't known, but now he was pain-free and relaxed and I was the one feeling uncomfortable.

He looked a bit like a pirate with his surgical eye patch as the consultants had been able to remove the balloon through his lid rather than his skull. What incredibly marvellous people! I genuinely could have kissed the surgeon who brought my happy boy back to me – although he was a hottie and I was single, so that might have contributed to the urge.

On that note, I had started dating again. When I left Mark, I had resigned myself to the fact that many men would be deterred by the prospect of dating any mother of two, let alone one in my situation with an eternal child. I wondered if anyone would be brave enough to take us on, but my boys were my priority and that was my focus.

Nevertheless, I found myself missing the company and intimacy of a relationship (i.e. I was lonely and sexually frustrated), so I was back in the terrifying dating arena where mind games, booty calls, fake profiles and horrendous yet hilarious disaster stories awaited. But here's the thing – when you have a child with special needs who relies on you completely, at what point do you mention him? To say nothing would feel like I was denying Harry's existence or was ashamed of his issues, which I wasn't at all, but it would give me a chance to spend some time getting to know a guy just as me. Charlene. Teacher and mum rather than permanently exhausted carer and decision maker of life for two. But it came with the risk that I might become attached to a guy and have to explain my situation only for it to be too much for him, and my fragile heart would be back on the shelf again.

The other option was to be upfront and to tell the guy right at the beginning. To explain that a life with me came with slightly more complications than most, but assure him that we were all worth it. To present him with a future he hadn't yet signed up to over a meal for two and a pint of Stella may mean that he would respect me, pity me or crap himself, thinking that I was looking for a father for my boys and already had a venue booked and a wedding dress on order. Yes, intense overthinking is one of my qualities.

In the end, I decided to be straight from the off. I registered with an online dating site as the idea of propping up a bar, hunting or being hunted and drunken chat-up lines filled me with dread. I explained that I was a mum of two children, one of whom had special needs, and was looking to make friendships with a view to seeing where they may lead.

I had a wide variety of responses, one from a young war veteran who also shared his story with pride and honesty, but who wanted explicit photos of me and described in detail what he would do with them. I didn't know whether to laugh or be sick in my mouth. There were other messages that burned my retinas and scarred me for life! A seemingly chatty and confident guy who met me for drinks turned out to be a painfully shy borderline selective mute. When I texted my girlfriends from the toilet and begged for help, they just laughed. And then there was a guy whose creepy message I deleted immediately, only to be bombarded by a torrent of abuse and vile promises of what he would do if he ever found me to get revenge. I wonder if he ever found love. In prison, maybe.

However, among the intense and insane were a few really nice guys. I dated two for a few months (not at the same time), but they didn't lead anywhere past the initial 'getting to know you' lust and giggles. Still, they were good while they lasted and boosted my self-esteem to a level it hadn't been for many years. I'm still friends with them on Facebook and love seeing the families and happiness they both went on to have.

On the whole, though, for the first part of 2011, Oliver, Harry and I were a happy trio. Just as I was resigning myself to staying that way for a while, a friend contacted me to say she knew of a great guy and asked if I would like to meet him. To be honest, I couldn't be bothered. I wasn't enjoying the emotional rollercoaster of the dating scene, but she assured me that he was a keeper and so I agreed at least to add him on Facebook – the 21st Century equivalent to foreplay – and investigate.

On Saturday 23 April, I visited some other friends who happened to invite out a single friend for me, but I knew early on in the night that there would be no romance with the lovely yet overly tactile chap. I lay in bed that night and wrote a list in the notes on my phone – a wish list describing the perfect man for the universe to receive and deliver on – and then I slept.

The following day, after a late and boozy night, another date was the last thing I wanted to put myself through, other than with my sofa and pyjamas. On the Sunday afternoon, I reluctantly took myself along to a local pub, determined to spend no more than three hours there, and was pleasantly surprised to be greeted by a guy who not only looked fairly normal, but was actually attractive. He didn't appear to have any pervy tendencies and wasn't a sexually frustrated octopus so the date went well.

So well, in fact, that we carried on talking over dinner and well into the night. Sunday 24 April 2011 was the day the universe responded to my list and I met Andrew, the love of my life, even though it turned out that he hadn't been enthusiastic about going along either and only went to keep our mutual friend quiet.

Fate is a funny thing.

Andrew and I spent the next three months getting to know each other without the distractions or complications of children. He was recently separated and had a young daughter and son whom he was fiercely protective of. His time with them was incredibly precious, and so we took things slowly.

Happy Days

I was still taking the boys to see Nicola, and her notes show that both had become very clingy since I had met Andrew. Harry continued to have an incredibly erratic sleep pattern despite my best efforts to introduce routine and structure, and he seemed even more keen to be close to me day and night. Meanwhile, Oliver was having phases of sleepwalking and climbing in bed with me to add to the sea of arms and legs. His self-esteem was still extremely low and he struggled to accept praise from me or my family for his fantastic mid-year school report. His breathing was shallow and laboured, his chatter was 100mph, and he was torn between loving his brother and feeling frustrated and isolated from him.

My boy was constantly vying for praise and attention that he somehow felt unworthy of. I don't know many adults who could cope with the loneliness that Oliver felt daily, and both Mark and I tried hard to reassure him that he was loved and treasured. He was worried about the house move as Mark prepared to sell our family home and could sense that there were tangible changes in his mummy's mood that he didn't understand. Even though these changes were good ones, maybe a part of him – the same part that knew we were moving out even before I had the chance to explain – knew that our trio was evolving.

It wasn't all bad. Oliver's character continued to develop and his personality shone through. Quick-witted, sarcastic and old-headed, he had us all in fits of laughter, often forgetting he was as young as he was. So much like me as a child. With a dad who is also chatty and sociable, Oliver was always going to be swimming in the personality-rich end of the gene pool. He wasn't a child prone to temper tantrums or strops – I think Harry had enough of that quality for them both – and his manners were impeccable. I was proud to take him anywhere as everyone commented on what a lovely boy he was.

In many ways, Harry's autism meant that he grasped concrete concepts such as phonic sounds and numbers very quickly, but Oliver struggled. Long before it was confirmed that he was dyslexic, I worked hard for him to know that no matter where he was in the class or the world, good manners were essential.

He crept downstairs one night in the May of 2011, just after I had put Harry to bed, which meant it was already quite late. I whispered, "Why are you still awake?" and he shushed me with his finger to his lips, climbed next to me and patted my cheek.

"Hush, little lady," he said. "I'll tell you when it's mission accomplished."

Stifling my giggles, I asked him what the mission was.

"Falling asleep with you, Mummy."

Being mad at that boy is impossible at times.

By the time my boys' sixth birthday arrived, in the June of 2011, I felt happier than I had done in a long time. At 10.30am – the precise time that the false announcement of "We've got two healthy boys" had disintegrated before us and we were plunged into shock and uncertainty – I watched the time pass without a tear for the first year since their birth. To say that my boys' birth day was the hardest of my life makes me incredibly sad, but it's true. So to be finally moving forward from that felt liberating.

I have to say that each year had been getting easier, the real life replay less vivid, but from here on I would feel only happiness and gratitude for both of my boys on their birthday. Much soul searching, many tears, hundreds of pounds in therapy and good old-fashioned time combined to make me a stronger version of the person I had always been and the mother I was destined to become.

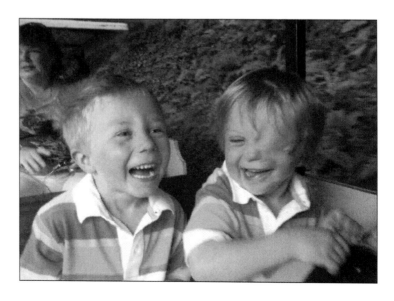

Bursts of Brilliance

I wasn't the only one making progress. Harry's speech was coming on beautifully. He was more tolerant when people struggled to understand him, and rather than losing his temper every time, he persevered until he could be understood, which was a massive achievement. He could be heard occasionally telling himself "Good job" in the American accent that Lisa used and he was taking part in more activities at school, declaring, "Finished now!" at the end.

At home, he used this new phrase to tell us when he'd had enough – enough food, enough waiting for his Nexus, or whenever we stopped him from doing something. Our attempts, according to Harry, would be "Finish now", and more than once he had us laughing out loud.

His willingness to communicate was also getting better, and one night he sat in the bath yelling, "Mummy! Mummy!" before thrusting foam letters into my hand and telling me a word beginning with each one.

"T is for 'urtle, Mummy."

He amazes me constantly.

The progress of a special needs child is unlike that of a 'typical' child. While Oliver grasps concepts gradually and regularly builds on prior knowledge, moving his understanding forward at a steady pace, Harry has spikes and plateaux. For months, he remains the same. Then all of a sudden, he will grasp a concept and dazzle and amaze us in the same way that most parents are astounded to see their child take their first steps. At any moment, a new behaviour, word or ability will present itself, often without warning, and suddenly it is us playing catch up with Harry. Those moments are exciting, wonderful and full of hope for a future that shows signs of potential.

And then it stops. If we are lucky, life stays the same for a while until the next burst of brilliance propels Harry forward again, but sometimes there is regression. Sometimes we take one step forward and three steps back. Instead of a waltz through life, it's more of a cha-cha, and yes, it is frustrating. But we never stop dancing.

One of Harry's many gifts is to take us by surprise in revealing that he is more present in a moment than he seems. Just because a child is non-verbal does not mean that they are not paying attention. One of my main pieces of advice to other parents would be never talk over the child's head as if they are not in the room. They may not be able to tell you they can hear you, but trust me, they can.

For years, I sang *Twinkle, Twinkle, Little Star* to Harry, only I changed the words.

"Mummy loves her little treasure,
Having him is such a pleasure,
Every day and every night,
She hopes she loves and treats him right.

Mummy loves her little boy,
He is such a pride and joy."

I sang it to him in the hope that he might join in, and one day, completely from nowhere, he did. He let me sing each line and sang the last couple of words with me.

When I had finished, he grinned his cheeky grin and demanded, "Mummy hand!" so that he could bend my fingers all the way back and make me yelp. To Harry, he was just singing along to the regular words he had heard for years. To me, he was letting me know that there was a way I could reach him. I must never give up hope and remember that none of my efforts went unnoticed.

The joy that filled a heart that had once ached so much was immense, and there are no words for how fiercely I wanted to wrap my arms around him and disappear into him. In those moments, to say I loved my boy just doesn't come close.

Three Become Six

In June, Andrew and I met each other's children, and for the next couple of months we had days out and evenings in just as 'friends'. Rather like teenagers sneaking around so that their parents didn't catch them snogging, we caught stolen moments over the bread bin when the children were playing. It was funny, exciting, and it was the right thing to do.

For both of us, our children were our priority. They had been through a lot. Andrew's children were still in the early stages of adjusting to separated parents so we believed that it was only fair to them to take things slowly. Our merry band of six spent time getting to know each other and learning to function as a unit, even though the children didn't realise it at the time.

For Harry, it made little difference. Benedicta and Harrison were just two more children for him to work around. He was now beginning to use other children if he wanted to get something in return. He would pass them a toy guitar and step back to bounce, indicating that he would like them to play and entertain him as if he were a medieval king. Which they did. Or he would lead them to a cupboard and push their hands towards the biscuits so that they would get some for him. I'm convinced his logic was that if they got caught, they'd get blamed. Again they complied and it was always far too amusing to be annoying.

His tantrums and outbursts took Andrew's children by surprise, whereas Oliver, like the seasoned veteran he was, carried on around the chaos, but generally they liked Harry, despite the fact that he rarely gave anything back. One of his many gifts is to make an unsuspecting acquaintance fall in love with him with a cute smile and a charming character.

But no one fell for Harry quite like Andrew did. Not only was he tolerant of Harry's behaviour and outbursts, but he supported him and tried hard to help with his frustrations. He also played with him as he did any other child (seriously, Andrew's like the Pied Piper, attracting a small gathering of boys and girls wherever he goes). Watching Andrew fall in love with Harry made me fall more in love with Andrew. The way to a man's heart may be through his stomach, but the way to a mother's heart is through her children, and it melted me like butter on hot toast to see Andrew not just accepting Harry, but appreciating and valuing him for the unique gift he is.

Oliver was enjoying having a man around the house again. Once we settled into a routine of boy night, girl night and a sprinkling of Andrew nights – sometimes on his own, sometimes with 'the kids' as Oliver still calls them six years later – he began to look forward to the variety of the week rather than being fearful of the uncertainty. He was loving having the company of children who actually played with him and talked to him, too.

We felt like a part-time family, so it was a natural transition, a few months after we had first introduced the children to each other, to tell them we were more than friends. They were thrilled, and life continued as it had – uninterrupted, safe and full of hope. Life was good.

The Fear vs The Faith

However, as is life, once we had come to rest, the impact of previous events hit us. Towards the end of 2011 something was changing again in me. This time it was a darkness.

It started slowly. On the advice of a friend of my mum's, whom I had been visiting for some incredible vortex sessions to work on my energy levels, I had been taking Rhodiola to level my mood. But my moods were becoming more intense. I could be driving to school either singing at the top of my voice and bouncing like Harry in my seat or choking on tears, physically unable to bear the sound of the radio. There was no pattern. There was no warning. Each night I went to bed unsure of how I would feel in the morning. Apprehensive about closing my eyes on the place I was in, only to wake into uncertainty.

Yet I smiled; of course I smiled. I laughed and I entertained, much like Oliver did. I performed. But it was all behind a mask. Increasingly I was feeling hollow and detached from myself again, a voyeur on a life that was confusing and exhausting.

I still wasn't sleeping particularly well on the nights the boys were with me. Divorce proceedings from the best friend I had married had begun and our home was being sold, so my new happy heart was also a bruised, heavy heart. Irrational thoughts meant that I regressed to a place of blame and shame for the first time in a long time. I began to wonder whether my boys would have a happier life without me in it. After all, I had caused so much heartache already. I questioned whether Mark could provide a life of financial security and emotional stability more than a manic crackpot who didn't know her own mind. Maybe they would be happier in the long run with him full-time.

Maybe on a Sunday, when the boys were with Mark and no one was expecting to see anything of me as I did my school work, I could just stay asleep. Forever. No drama. No horrendous scenes for the person who tried to wake me. Just sleeping Charlene. The thought flew around my brain like a dog chasing its tail. Relentlessly.

But there were two things that kept me here and awake. Two reasons not to quit on life just yet. Two little people worth fighting my demons for. Ironically, it was the same love for my boys that made me think I would be helping them if I was no longer here that saved me from leaving their side.

In the end, I confided in my mum that all was not as it appeared. That I felt I was lost and sinking, but I couldn't give up on a life I had worked so hard on and I needed some help. My mum cuddled me, her broken baby, in the same way all parents do with their precious little ones and said that we needed to see the doctor. She took me to discuss my situation with the professionals, who asked me a series of questions. I nodded without looking up, hunched over and bitterly ashamed. Feeling weak and pathetic that my life had got to this point, I left with what I hoped would be sunshine in a bottle and a regular review appointment set up to monitor me.

Two years later, I wrote the following in the hope that one day someone would read it and it would help them.

*****

The Fear vs The Faith
There is nothing more terrifying than not knowing your own mind. Not knowing whether you will wake ready to face the world or whether you'll truly believe it's a better place without you, be paralysed by this conviction, and unable to get out of bed. So, two years ago, I allowed myself to be taken to the doctors. I sat hunched and crying, defeated and ashamed as my mum explained that her daughter needed saving from herself.

I had always believed that antidepressants were for the weakest victims and I cried every night for a while as I took mine. But very slowly, my darkness left me. There were no hysterical outbursts of laughter or spontaneous jazz hands and cartwheels as I had feared. Just balance and calm. Clarity and strength. And ever so slowly, I began to believe in myself again and not fear what the next day would bring.

Two years later I had come to appreciate the value of my crutch and the old fear was replaced by a new one: how would I ever cope without the antidepressants? So I weaned myself off medicated balance and back into reality. Unstable, unpredictable reality. But I did it, and I want everyone who is as terrified and lost as I was to know that they can too.

Do I still believe that antidepressants are a sign of weakness? Absolutely not! Would I go back on them if I felt that I needed to? In a heartbeat. And there lies the strength and the peace: knowing that we're not superhuman and that sometimes we do need support to get us through the next mission to save the world (or do the weekly shop). Acknowledging this is the hardest and the bravest thing I've ever done, but I've done it. And so can you X.

Options

Once I had adjusted to the medication – both mentally and physically – life calmed. My mood became more stable and I was able to enjoy a life which was rich with love from both my boys and Andrew.

This was great timing as the appointment came through at Alder Hey to discuss the next steps for Harry. Had the balloon not caused any problems, Harry may not have had more surgery for a couple of years, but the surgeons now had up-to-date scans to refer to and felt that the time was right to consider our options.

Mark and I went along and listened as they explained what they felt to be our choices. The first was to do nothing. As none of Harry's surgery was in response to a life-threatening condition, this was always an option. However, as always, we wrestled with the prospect of (a) leaving Harry untouched by surgery but maybe emotionally damaged by an unforgiving society, or (b) having the operations in the hope that he could live a life without judgement or bullying. For the man-child Harry would become, one day living without us here, we felt doing nothing was not an option this time.

Harry's CT scans had revealed that the front of his skull was slightly too far pronounced, meaning that his brain was filling a gap that shouldn't be there. This needed to be corrected at the same time as creating a new eye socket, but so much was unknown. The staff at Alder Hey were still working with the remnants of the previous attempt at a socket, so although they had a plan, until they took his skull apart they wouldn't fully see what they were dealing with.

Taking his skull apart. I felt sick.

We chatted about the craniotomy procedure, the bone grafting that would be required and the soft tissue that would need to be taken from elsewhere in his body and donated to the birth of an eye socket. We talked at length about the operation, what would be involved, the risks and the degree of uncertainty about the outcome. I should have been terrified by this, and a part of me was, but based on the fact that the team had consulted with us at every stage, always been straight with us and never offered false promises, I trusted their judgement. I hoped and prayed that my trust wasn't misplaced for a second time.

We talked about the socket that Harry would have and the further operations to create an eyelid. If, for some reason, an ocular prosthesis (false eye) was not possible, then there were options of facial prostheses to consider, but all decisions would stem from the first operation and we wouldn't know until it had been completed. Like pushing the first domino over and watching each one behind it fall in turn, we knew the impact of that operation would be huge, but it had to be done. It was both exciting and terrifying to feel that things were changing for us all again, but we believed we were placing Harry in good hands.

Never a Dull Moment

Oliver has always had a cheeky smile and an endearing sense of mischief, but as he grew older, his sense of humour and little insights had me in stiches. In doing my research to document our journey, I saw from my Facebook status updates that 2012 was the year my son was one gag away from becoming a stand-up comedian, not in a deliberate attention-seeking way, but in a natural, dry, observational way that to this day makes him seem older than his years and loved by his audiences.

Like the evening we sat together, watching the latest *Dance Competition*. One of the judges, Kimberley Wyatt, congratulated an incredible pole dancer on her feet, legs, lines and strength, at which point Oliver piped up, "And she's *smokin'* hot! *Enchanté*," with a wink, "grrrrrrrrr!" I wondered whether I should worry about his healthy appreciation of the female form at his age.

On another evening, he told me over dinner that I was looking super sexy and he was going to smooch with me once we had finished.

"Are you?" I asked.

He actually *smouldered* at me and said, "Yeah, you're dessert. Grrrr!" and then we both burst into fits of laughter.

Another time, he decided to give me image advice. "Mummy, if Andrew ever dumps you, you should have your hair all messy like you've just got out of bed, wear a black, *not pink*, biker jacket and dark red lipstick, and always remember, men love women who are powerful, and girls love a bad boy."

Seriously? Where did he get it all from? He was hilarious.

One evening he called me from his dad's and I told him that I was missing him. He told me that he was missing me too. I told him that I loved him. He replied that he loved me more. I reminded him that he was the very best son in the word.

He said, "I know."

His natural way with people and the ease with which he initiated or joined conversations with others, often adults, would have fooled many into believing that Oliver was an incredibly confident child, but behind the bravado he lacked a true sense of self-worth. I met with the school special needs worker who had assessed him for dyslexia to be told that I had an incredibly charming and articulate son destined for the stage, but he had a chronically low self-image as a learner. This made me proud yet so sad, and I wished then, as I do now, that he could see the incredible boy he is both inside and outside of the classroom. I love him more fiercely every day.

Harry, of course, was spared such turmoil. Throughout his life, he has been blissfully unaware of the obstacles he faces; the challenges; the natural comparisons with classmates; where he sits in the social and academic league table with his peers. One of the few silver linings to the cloud of Harry's conditions is that he has escaped constant inner-evaluation and appraisal. He is free from it all, and in that respect, he is more fortunate than most.

However, this also means that he does not understand the rules and pressures of things like social acceptance and academic performance. More than once, Oliver and I have had heated discussions about the need for him to complete his reading, spellings or homework. As Oliver gets so frustrated and reluctant to engage in the things which make him feel inadequate that he cries and shouts, Harry finds it absolutely hilarious. He giggles, which then turns into a full-blown laughing fit. As soon as he has had enough entertainment, he will either walk away or push Oliver over to silence him. I shouldn't laugh, but it's hard not to.

Then I think that maybe Harry's behaviour adds to Oliver's frustrations. Back to Guilt Central for me.

Harry often has phases of new fascinations which irritate and amuse me in equal measure. Removing the imitation coals from the electric fire and using them to write, like chalk, all over his clothes, toys and the carpets was one of his favourite games for a while. He also made a game from taking anything made of paper – my school books, thankfully, were never victims – and putting it into the washing machine on a 30 degree cycle while he bounced, clapped and flapped his arms furiously. He discovered that the microwave made a pinging noise when you pressed the button and a hissing noise with a touch of fireworks when he put something into it that shouldn't be there.

For a while he had a fascination with the slight indent ridges left by a sock around a person's ankle and would investigate the lower legs of all visitors to the house. To his credit, he widened this fascination to include the marks left by the waistband of jogging pants, but while it was the norm for him to lift my top and feel the ridges of the sportswear around my waist, the young girl on the monkey bars at Lulworth Castle wasn't quite so understanding when he dashed over to pull her trousers down. It's at times like these that I am grateful that Harry looks so different as unnerved parents calm more quickly when they see a visible explanation for his behaviour. I see the hypocrisy in hating people staring at his differences yet being relieved that he has them when it spares him the lynch mob, but if there are going to be any benefits for Harry looking so unique, this is probably one of my favourites.

Harry loves a reaction. Screaming, squealing or any kind of raised emotion is enough to reduce him to a giggling wreck. Parents chastising their children in Asda? Harry's laughing *and* pointing (earth, please swallow me up). Tread on some Lego and howl like you've lost a limb? Yep, Harry is rolling around on the floor. Trip up the stairs carrying armfuls of toys and swear like a trooper? Harry is still at the bottom of the stairs, laughing hard.

I sat at the side of Harry's bath one night, listening to a voicemail message. It was from Oliver, saying, "Mummy, I got my 10 metres badge at swimming. Are you proud of me? You're always proud of me, mwah!" As I smiled, listening to my boy's happy voice, Harry filled his mouth with water and spat it all over me, delighted by my sudden squeal and jump into the air. There was never a dull moment.

And the fun continued through the night.

Nocturnal Visitors

When my boys were five weeks old, the Special Care nurse who had done a night shift with them told me, "That one loves eating," Oliver, "and that one just wants to be cuddled all night," Harry. And it appears that each infant at five weeks was a pretty good indicator of the children they would be aged seven.

I tried, unsuccessfully, many times to return Harry to his own bed when he bounded into mine, full of energy. Harry got the same amount of rest and recharging in three hours that most people require seven to achieve and so it was difficult to settle him down again. He would wander downstairs, and the first I would know of him being awake would be a musical interlude blaring from the lounge or the thud of his toys being thrown repeatedly against the adjoining neighbours' wall, so I would leap out of bed and join him on the sofa.

Sometimes he would bring several toys to my bed and hit 'play' at the same time so I was jolted awake at 1.30am by a synchronised VTech frenzy of lights and tunes. I was conscious that he was waking not only me, but also Oliver, so at times when I was on my own, I would pull him into bed with me just to keep him quiet. This didn't always work, and more than once, Oliver fell asleep in class or cried about being tired from the nocturnal goings on at home.

Harry just wanted company, and I understood this. I actually liked cuddling him in my bed, his little arms around my neck and his soft face on mine, but I knew that if I didn't stop him from doing this, the eternal child within him would still be trying to climb into bed with me when he was a 25-year-old man.

He had the box room at the front of the house, which had the soft lighting and calming environment that Lisa had recommended, but he wanted a body next to him. Once Andrew started to stay over some nights, this became hard to manage. I tried, as I had done before, to return Harry to his own bed. Several times a night. Often I would imagine the *Benny Hill* music playing as I dived over my bed to grab him before he jumped in, or took his arm to frogmarch him back to his own room. I could do that four or five times each night.

Sometimes I sat on the floor until he settled; sometimes I just put him into bed and walked out; occasionally I held the door shut behind me while he banged and shouted for me to open it again, which I did very quickly on account of the fact that he would wake Oliver and I felt like a wicked mother. Sometimes, usually the fourth or fifth attempt, I would lie with him, telling myself that I would get up again shortly then waking the next morning, feeling exhausted and sick even before my day of teaching 30 children had begun.

It was relentless. If I got up eight times with Harry, he had a ninth attempt in him. More often than not,

Harry won – catching up on his sleep during a power nap on the school transport. If I had a pound for every time I wished I had his superpowers for reenergising, I would have retired already.

My friend had a genius idea of putting a blow-up camp bed on the floor next to me, and for a while, Harry liked the novelty. But he still had to be touching some part of me. His little voice in the darkness would demand, "Mummy hand!" and I would feel like I was dislocating my right shoulder to drop my hand to where he lay. Sometimes I managed to fool him with 'Mummy foot' by lying upside down in my bed and hanging my left leg out for him to touch, but that didn't last long. He would have the hand.

As soon as I could hear his rhythmic snuffling breathing, I would return all of my body parts to bed to warm up, only for him to ask for them again a couple of hours later. And regardless of the battles we had throughout the night, I was usually a human trampoline from around 4.30am anyway.

Sometimes, Harry would be sleeping and *Oliver* would wander in, dazed and confused. My dilemma here was whether to clamber over Sleeping Beauty to return Oliver to his own bed, running the risk of waking Harry, or silently beckon Oliver to the other side of the bed, despite not allowing Harry the same luxury. It was a tough one, but I was exhausted, so more often than not, Oliver would join me.

Oliver was still massively insecure and nervous about me not being with him, and some mornings I would find him asleep on the landing carpet outside my door.

"Just so I'd know if you left in the night, Mummy," he'd say.

My only respite was the nights when the boys stayed with Mark. You would think that I would naturally fall into a deep sleep, but it appeared that my body was now wired for regular interruptions and so I woke anyway, sometimes hearing the noises of boys who weren't even there. Those were the nights when I needed a glass of rosé wine and a super-powerful antihistamine so that I could capture the sleep which had eluded me for so long.

All of this was slowly playing havoc with my sanity and health, and so, with Harry's operation rapidly approaching, I took the difficult decision to request my teaching contract be reduced to part-time hours. I knew that this would give me some time to myself where my body could rest and recharge, but I also knew that a teacher like me, who was passionate about high standards of learning and took the responsibility for the social, emotional and educational development of my class very seriously, would find a job share hard. My head teacher knew this too, and warned me that I would be trading one problem for another. But I physically couldn't carry on as I had done, and so 2012 was my last year as a full-time teacher.

A New Home

I was making some changes on the home front, too. Our old family home was in the final stages of being sold, and I had spotted a 1930s semi-detached house for sale just up the road from where we were. Its owner had moved into a retirement home, so when I viewed it, it was an empty shell of a once well-loved family home. I fell in love with it, too.

It needed a lot of work to bring it up to date – electrics, plumbing, a new bathroom suite and kitchen, full plastering and decorating, as well as a wall being totally knocked down, but I saw the potential there. It had no immediate neighbours other than its mirror image attached twin, and a fantastic sized lawn around three sides. It also had a single-storey garage, and as I considered the scale of the project, I was filled with excitement at the thought of replacing it with a two-storey extension that Harry could call home in his later years so that he would never have to live in sheltered accommodation.

Harry's future was, and still is, at the forefront of many of the decisions I've made for our lives. Oliver will probably move into his own family home one day, but Harry doesn't have the same freedom of choice, and so I am always considering the future I can help shape for Harry. For those of us who have a unique child to consider, the impact on our collective tomorrows of the decisions we make today is something that not many people grasp. I certainly wouldn't have considered it had Mark and I had the life we were expecting. So when I explained my rationale for buying a property which was probably far too big for me, even my nearest and dearest were taken aback. They had never considered Harry's future beyond the next few years.

People don't. Even the most well-meaning, helpful and amazing of them don't see it like we do: the huge ever-present reminder of responsibility; the insurance policy and risk assessment for a life that should have been ordinary, but is entirely extraordinary. At first, it felt lonely to know that no one instinctively got the fact that my brain is thinking about life 20 years from now when I make a big decision, or even three hours from now when I plan to go out with the family. The constant processing of what needs to be done to make sure that everyone enjoys the day while juggling the emotions of a child who struggles in unfamiliar places.

But now, I kind of like that it's just me. In my head, I defend and uphold my right as Harry's protector. Gone are the days when I worried about coping and questioned whether I was up to the job of being Harry's mum. It's now my greatest pleasure to be the mum of both my boys, and my mission is to ensure that Harry lives as full a life as he can. I don't know when that transformation occurred. Probably very slowly through the years, but I am thankful every day that it did.

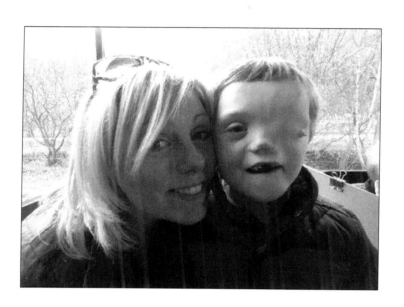

Difficult Lessons

Andrew and I took the children away for a long weekend to a caravan in Wales. Harry loved the fresh air and the freedom of wandering over the sand dunes without me holding him by the wrist – autistic children have a tendency to slip out of a hand grasp. It was also amazing to see Oliver become more relaxed, and he strayed further and further away from me with Benedicta and Harrison as his guides.

One afternoon, the three of them decided to follow me to the onsite store. Harry wanted to go with them, but Andrew explained that he had to wait. The others were just going to the shop and they wouldn't be long.

Now, to most children that would make sense, but to Harry, 'shop' meant Toys R Us. 'Shop' was the equivalent to the big red button being pressed just before a NUC gets fired. And Harry was fired. He kicked, fought and scratched.

By the time we walked back from the shop, I could hear him screaming and dashed to the caravan. Andrew was distraught and had no idea what had brought on Harry's behaviour. When I heard what he had said and explained the significance of the word 'shop', he was devastated. Just one word, used correctly and innocently but filled with a different kind of meaning for Harry, had reduced him to a wreck.

Eventually he sobbed himself to sleep in my arms, but even then, through his sleep he gasped and whimpered. It was weeks before he returned to his Andrew-loving self, and it was an incredibly difficult lesson for Andrew as he bravely took on the world of special needs where words, routines or actions hold so much power.

*****

My boys' seventh birthday party was great. We held it in the village hall with all of Oliver's friends as I didn't know Harry's friends. He couldn't come home and tell me about his day; he didn't share stories of who he had played with or fallen out with. I knew nothing of the challenges that his peers faced. My only communication with school was through his home school diary. I wouldn't have recognised any of his classmates like I knew Oliver's, and I think that some part of me was embarrassed by that.

And so, rather than ask parents or think of a creative way to find out each child's name when they arrived, I just didn't invite them. Harry would be quite content to bounce and giggle with Oliver's friends, who loved him anyway. Sometimes, looking back, you see where you could have done so much more, but hindsight is 20/20 and I refuse to beat myself up for the mistakes I made while I was trying my best.

The Cruelty of Ignorance

Harry's operation was rapidly approaching. Mark and I had met with the surgeons a couple of times since our initial chat and were aware of the risks they were incredibly keen to stress to us. If, when they removed the front of Harry's skull, any of the arteries from his brain that had been pressing against the bone were to tear, there could be bleeding on the brain, the results of which they couldn't predict. But the risks of this were negligible compared to the results that the surgeons were confident they could achieve.

The date was set for 2 July 2012, and we were counting down to a date that filled us with both fear and hope. Oliver was nervous. He would cry and tell me that he didn't want his brother's face to change, that he loved Harry as he was. Those conversations were so hard, but when we were out and about, faced with discrimination and cruelty, Oliver understood.

It made me sad that my six-year-old had to see the dark side of human nature so young; that he should experience the rage of a protective brother and sorrow of empathy. It was a learning journey for us all, and I hated that I couldn't spare Oliver from those parts. Like the sunny afternoon I took my boys with Nan to the local park. A group of boys, there without parents, decided to shout obscenities at Harry, laugh, point and tease him, and then follow us as we cut our trip short to walk around the lake instead. I was seething inside, and yes, I had some choice words for them which made them snarl at me before shrugging and walking away. I visualised myself punching every one of those children in the face. My adrenalin raced as I pummelled, kicked and thrashed them in my mind, releasing years of repressed rage, but I knew that if I laid so much as a finger on a child, I would lose my job as a teacher. I took a deep breath and we went home, all of us drained (except Harry, who bounced regardless).

So when Oliver questioned why Harry needed his operations, I reminded him of the cruelty of those boys and that I wouldn't always be there to protect his brother.

And Oliver said, "I understand now. Thank you, Mummy. I love you."

Sunshine Boy

I finished school for the summer with an incredible send-off of flowers, chocolates – typical teacher gifts – and a hospital hamper of sweets, magazines, mints, dry shampoo and Femfresh. Before we knew it, the day of the operation was upon us.

I lay on the bed with Harry, waiting for the nurses to take us to theatre. Harry was the first case on the list with the expectation of a six-hour operation, and Mark was dropping Oliver off at school before racing to us, but as that day began it was just me and my boy. We played with his toys, we watched *Peppa Pig* on the TV and we cuddled. I lay at his right side and pulled him close to me so I could rest my cheek on his head. I stroked his hair and his little face. I inhaled his smell like he was a bouquet of flowers and I sang to him.

"You are my sunshine, my only sunshine,
You make me happy, when skies are grey.
You'll never know, dear, how much I love you.
Please don't take my sunshine away."

Three different members of staff came to check that I had read the consent form and was aware of the risks.

The last time they asked, I said, "Yes, but if you ask me again, I'll change my mind!" My heart was racing, my throat was aching from holding the massive lump of terror there, and I was hyper-sensitive to every part of my boy – his voice, his skin, his kisses.

It felt like eternity until I finally took him to theatre. I stayed as he wrestled slightly with the mask to sedate him; I kissed the very forehead that would be lying in a sterile tray within a few hours and told him that I loved him and would see him soon. I cried as I left him and asked my grandad to take care of my sunshine boy.

Mark joined me in the cafeteria where I was trying to eat, but struggling. It had only been an hour since I had left Harry, but I watched the clock and the time dragged painfully. We drank coffees and chatted, read magazines, made phone calls to our families with updates we didn't have and waited.

After six hours, we returned to the ward and waited in the communal parents' room where we stared at a TV screen full of afternoon randomness and saw none of it. I began to read *Handle with Care* by Jodi Picoult, never expecting just one paragraph to change something in me so profoundly that I would never be the same mum again. The main character in the story talks of her life with her disabled daughter.

> *Other people look at me and think: That poor woman; she has a child with a disability. But all I see when I look at you is that girl who had memorized all the words to* Queen's Bohemian Rhapsody *by the time she was three, the girl who crawls into bed with*

me whenever there's a thunderstorm – not because you're afraid but because I am, the girl whose laugh has always vibrated inside my own body like a tuning fork. I would never have wished for an able-bodied child, because that child would have been someone who wasn't you.

Jodi Picoult, *Handle with Care*

In that exact moment I thought about all the things that Harry did. His little quirks. The things that annoyed and amused me. The constant bouncing until the springs in my sofa and bed were exhausted and protesting in squeaks. His incessant demands for batteries so that he could replace perfectly good ones with even better ones the second his hyper-sensitive ear heard the power begin the fade. The pain of him grabbing my hand to bend the fingers right back and explore my palm. The inappropriate laughing; the nocturnal antics. The way he nuzzled into my neck when I picked him up. How he clung to me like a monkey with his legs wrapped around my waist and refused to be lowered to the ground. The way he insisted on grabbing my cheeks and pulling me to face him in bed, the sickly sweet smell of catarrh breath wafting my way.

All of those things weren't just what Harry did, they were who Harry was. If he hadn't been born the way he had, then he wouldn't have been Harry. He would have been an entirely different person and not the boy I loved with every breath in my body. That paragraph shifted something in me so much that I cried. Even now, years later, when I have a moment where I feel sorry for myself and frustrated with our lives, I think of it and in an instant, I feel better. One paragraph set one part of me free forever.

*****

After seven hours, we began to worry. The operation should have been done by now, and as much as people said no news was good news, we wanted some either way.

I asked the staff to call theatre and ask, but they only said the surgeons were still working on him and had nothing more to give us. If the first seven hours dragged, the remaining three-and-a-half were positively excruciating.

Ten-and-a-half hours after I'd kissed my boy goodbye, he came back to the ward. He was heavily sedated and wore a turban of bandages, but the surgeons were thrilled with how it had all gone. They had actually been able to achieve more than they had expected. It really didn't matter to me what they had done to him at that point, though – I was just delighted to have him back with us.

A New Face

Over the next few days, Harry continued to show us all how brave and strong he was. The day after the operation, as the sedatives wore off, Harry realised that his only eye had swollen closed. Temporarily, he was unable to see a thing, so I chatted with him and put toys in his hands to explore. He was unusually quiet, except for the odd 'ow' and request for 'ome, and I wished I could speed up his recovery. The only time I left his side was to shower, pee and eat, and then Mark was with him.

The staff were fantastic, but as much as Harry was making some great progress with his speech, those who didn't know him still required a translator. I stayed at his side, even when it meant I slept in an upright chair, because that's what we do. That's who we are, those of us who love, fight for and protect our unique children. Wrapping them in a shield of love and strength is our superpower.

As Harry's sight returned and his patience reduced, I took him to the ward toy room to explore some new toys. What I realised over those few days was just how few resources there actually were. The toys were fine but few; the felt-tip pens were dry or running out; the games console had been stolen; the DVDs were limited to a few cartoons and animated films – no good for the older children at all. And so I sent a message to my Facebook community, initially for donations of DVDs. I wanted to give something back to the staff who were looking after us so well and the other children and families who never chose to be on that ward, but smiled regardless.

I felt so relieved to have made the right decision for Harry. His new face was amazing, with bumps and dips in the right places, and his previous 'bud' of eyelids, which had protruded from his face with the balloon below, now turned inside out so that he had a slim and tidy permanent 'wink' instead. He wore a fresh zigzagging 'pumpkin-style' scar over the top of his head from ear to ear, and he smiled at me every day.

After just eight days, the surgeons said that Harry was well enough to go home. We left with jubilant hearts, knowing that a better future and over 100 DVDs for the hospital were waiting for us.

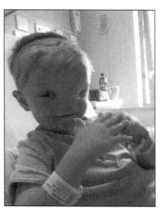

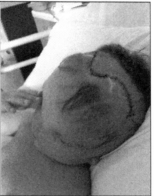

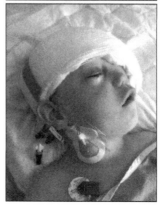

Fundraising and Fame

Raising awareness of the need for more DVDs and equipment for the hospital soon turned into raising money so the ward staff could purchase new items themselves. A race night was organised with the fantastic help of Clare and Darren, who did fundraisers for various causes and charities. I contacted the local newspaper which ran a great article on the event and my mission to encourage people to donate money and prizes.

The race night was a huge success. Seeing so many friends pull together to help me in my quest was touching and amazing. Mark brought both boys along to make a guest appearance, and the people who had donated their time, effort and money were even more motivated to make the night a great success after they had witnessed the boys' magical charisma. The evening raised just over £2,000 and I was elated! Three months of planning, stressing and worrying had all been worth it.

A few weeks later, I received a phone call from an agent in Manchester called Lucy who had seen the local publicity and wanted to write a longer article in *Woman's Own* magazine. She also wanted to represent me and the boys in terms of any other publicity that might be offered. It had never occurred to me that people who didn't know us would be interested in our story, but then I thought of the article I had read at the hairdressers, many years earlier, of a mother's unconditional love and instant bonding with her special needs child, and the very different experience that I'd had. I agreed and Lucy interviewed me over the phone.

We went to Manchester to have professional photographs taken by Gary, Lucy's husband, and made a day of it with my friends Sophie and Kate, exploring some museums there. Well, Oliver explored. Harry had several tantrums, but was contained enough for Oliver to enjoy the visit.

The photos of my boys were stunning and I felt incredibly proud of them. I supplied pictures that we had taken ourselves of our new-borns, and when the article was published it was so strange to see them in print. All the world could look at those photos, while I knew they were tucked safely away in an album under my stairs.

The article was beautifully written, and I dared to hope that another mother would draw comfort from my honest but hopeful account of an unexpected life. My family and friends loved it and the support was incredible. Soon, other magazines got in touch – *Pick Me Up*, *Chat* – and then the *Sun* newspaper and *Daily Mirror* online.

It was interesting, encouraging and soul-crushing in equal measures to read the comments left below my article online once it went viral. Some questioned what sort of mother could doubt her own love; one man commented that I should have aborted Harry;

others, mainly in America, said that I should have my children taken off me as I was a wicked person. As much as I understood that from the outside, it looked like I was cruel and uncaring, I knew that somewhere, some mother would be feeling the same, suffering in silence.

The few negative comments were drowned by the hundreds of supportive and positive messages of thanks and hope. It lifted my heart to think that I was helping anyone at all. Two years later, I received a random friend request from a lady who had been looking for me on social media but had struggled because I didn't use my married name to stop my pupils finding me. Her daughter had also been born with a very rare cranio-facial syndrome, and she didn't know anyone with anything similar in her city in Australia. It's a friendship I still have now and it is incredibly valuable to us both.

After the newspaper articles came a call to say that *Breakfast TV* wanted me and the boys to appear. I deliberated over the scale of what had grown from a local fundraiser article, but what was the point of being passionate about helping other people who might be feeling lost if I didn't follow it through?

Mark was unconvinced. He felt that it was exploiting the children for money and didn't see why it was so important to me that I did this. I informed him that we were being paid nothing other than travel expenses and reminded him of the wreck I had been in the early months after the boys had arrived. I asked him to remember how painful that was for us all, and explained that I hoped to save just one person from going through the same by offering some hope and honesty. Reluctantly, he agreed.

I spoke to the boys, too, informing them of what may happen. I have always explained to Harry what is happening, never talking over his head or presuming he can't hear or understand me. There is a pure wisdom inside my boy, far greater than anything outside of him, and so I explained where we would be going and why it was important to me.

Less heartfelt explanations were required with Oliver. As soon as he realised we'd be staying in a hotel with room service like *Home Alone 2*, he packed his pants and socks and was counting down the days. He was one excited boy.

And so the boys, the irritating ball machine and I, with my sister Emily along for the ride, set off for our TV debut in London.

Wishing upon a Star

The experience was fantastic. Although I have no recollection of what I said on camera, my phone was on fire with positive comments afterwards. Lucy contacted me again after that about a Japanese company which made short documentaries entitled *Miraculous People*, but when I did my research I found that it was tagged on to the end of a home movie calamity TV show. That was not the forum that I wanted. So, contrary to the speculation that I had put my children through the 'ordeal' of national television to make loads of money, I declined the first financially impressive but morally uncomfortable offer.

A few weeks after we held the race night, I received a call from a charity called When You Wish Upon A Star. We had a mutual friend who had donated some prizes to the evening and had told the charity about the cause. As much as we don't like to acknowledge it too much, we are a family with a child who has a life-limiting condition, and the charity supports families like ours to make memories and enjoy precious time together.

We were invited to Center Parcs for a week of activities and fun, and we were overwhelmed. The week was incredible with everything paid for, food included, and a themed evening which was like some kind of make-believe land. It was the only time I have heard Oliver be grateful for the fact that Harry has his disabilities, and although I cringed to think that Oliver was thrilled to be enjoying a 'freebie' off the back of our situation, I knew that he, more than any of us, deserved it.

He and Harry grew closer during that week when he was proud to show off his brother to the other families who totally understood and accepted the tantrums, the screams and the random outbursts. The peace of a week without the need to explain our life was bliss. To all be together, laughing and smiling regardless of the operations, appointments, stares and questions that waited for us outside of that bubble, was absolutely priceless. I can't even begin to imagine what it cost to organise, and we have since done some fundraising to give a little bit back. We will always be grateful to and supportive of this charity which has continued to give us amazing experiences at Hogwarts via the Orient Express and touring with its representatives to show its sponsors the value of the work that it does.

But by a mile, the most important thing I took away from that week is that we are not alone. There are so many families like ours, and so many families in even worse situations with children who will never reach adulthood, never walk or enjoy the simple pleasures that even my family takes for granted. I remind myself of them on the days when I feel low, tired or lost, and I remain in touch today with some of the families we met there.

Harry's next operation was scheduled for early September of the same year. We came home from Center

Parcs on a high, ready to face the next in a series of operations that will take Harry into his adulthood. This time it was to create the socket for his eventual prosthetic eye. Creating the socket was only one part of the process as it also needed to be lined.

After much discussion between consultants about where the skin grafts should be taken from, it was decided to remove them from the insides of Harry's mouth to create a 'wet' socket as opposed to the 'dry' one that skin from his thigh would create. And so on 9 September, I kissed Harry goodbye again and left him in the hands of the surgeons I now trusted completely.

After Harry's surgery, the staff in theatre rang the ward to say that 'Harry's parent' could go down to recovery to collect him, and off I skipped (not literally) to hold my boy again. However, when I got there, Harry was not as I had expected. He was lying on his right side with a bandage and patch over his left eye. His mouth was covered in blood which was already dark burgundy and congealed around the corners of his mouth and his teeth. His pillow was wet with saliva and he was gargling on his own blood as he breathed.

I went faint. The room swayed and I clung to the rail at the side of his bed to steady myself. He looked as if he had been in the most horrific fight of his life.

At that point, I heard that it was *Hallie* who was ready and waiting for her parents and not Harry. Of course, he was cleaned up in no time, and all that I had seen was part of the procedure. But seeing my child lying in his own blood made me question whether I was right to put him through it all. It was a question I asked with every appointment, every procedure and operation, but

I rationalised it as preparing my boy for the days when I wouldn't be around to protect him or be his voice. The day when the funny looking arm-flapping boy stopped being cute and became the awkward adult people laughed at or teased. Even now, the thought of that reality horrifies me, but I push it away and take one day at a time. It's like your satnav warning of hazards ahead, and you trusting that by the time you reach that point on your journey, they will have been resolved. Hope. It's all any of us have.

*****

Once Harry's bandages were removed, they revealed a full socket (amazing) which was filled with a bright green lump (weird). I didn't mean to sound ungrateful, but questioned whether there was a possibility of him having a slightly more discreet mould in the socket. It turns out that after much trial and error with other patients, the surgeons found that dental putty was the only material good enough to use, and as this was a lovely shade of pea, we were stuck with it. But we didn't care. Harry had the beginning of a socket and we dared to imagine what an eye would look like further down the road.

That road turned out to be the scenic route, and over the next two months we did the 120-mile round trip to the hospital a further nine times for various mishaps, adjustments, updates and lessons on inserting the mould into the newly formed socket. Not one for the squeamish or faint-hearted!

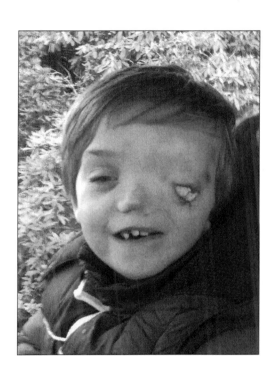

Awards for my Boys

At school, Harry was moving into Key Stage Two. Although he was unable to chat with me about his day and activities, I knew that he wasn't happy. He was agitated when it came to putting on his uniform and generally more grizzly. I'd expected some issues as his familiar staff and classroom changed, but I knew in my heart that he was sad in a way he couldn't express. As much as his new teacher was lovely, he was missing Lisa.

Of course, there was nothing we could do about the fact that he was growing older. He needed to move on, but it was hard for him. I felt helpless at his frustration and concerned when he started to fall behind in his skills, but by Christmas he was settling well. Nan and I applauded heartily as he made a very convincing World War II evacuee in his school Christmas concert. Nan had never missed a year and always lit up when her little man appeared.

If I had known that year would be her last, I would have taken so many more photographs.

*****

Often, when I tell people about Harry's conditions, they ask, "And is the other twin OK?" and I say he is fine but he's had his struggles in other ways. Harry's noisy nocturnal protests affected Oliver as well as us. For a while, Harry attempted to connect with his brother via the medium of a toy thrown at Oliver's head. And Oliver's cries made Harry laugh.

Although to Harry this was a game and his form of interaction, for Oliver it was torture and cruel. The brother who'd once ignored him now only communicated through hurting him. Oliver didn't sleep well, he didn't like himself, and he battled with so much outside of what was going on with Harry.

I knew that he was dyslexic long before any professionals confirmed it, and for a time he wore a built up shoe and endured several physiotherapy sessions to support a limp caused by one leg being marginally shorter than the other. This affected his balance and co-ordination, and to this day he can't walk down the stairs without putting both feet on one step at a time.

Yet despite all this, Oliver was doing well at school, too. What he lacked in mobility and self-belief he made up for in resilience and charisma. For his final year of first school, he was the recipient of the Rebecca Harris Trophy, given to one pupil each year for overcoming adversity. After the year Harry had had and the support that Oliver had given him, it had been a unanimous choice.

My nan and I attended the assembly as a surprise, and Oliver's face when he was announced as the winner was priceless. To see him have a moment of glory and recognition was incredible and melted my heart. The local newspaper was there to capture the moment and Oliver was thrilled to be the centre of attention for a while. He treasured the enormous trophy for the year that it was his.

A few months after Oliver received his award, I received a phone call from the same local newspaper, the *Sentinel*, to say that it would like to nominate Harry for its Child of Courage Award for 2014. I was stunned and agreed to some photographs and a short article to explain how proud I was of my boy and share his story. After our spate of magazine interviews, Harry was quite the poser for the photographer.

During the interview, I was asked which words I would use to describe Harry and gave them 'mischievous, energetic, determined, brave, loving and lovable'. When asked what the future held for Harry, I found that one a little harder. In a flash I could see all the things he might never do or have.

But I simply replied, "The future is unknown, but if someone had asked me eight years ago when he was born what his future would be like, I don't think I'd have imagined him achieving as much as he has now. So although it's unknown, it's also full of possibilities. He's a determined boy, so if he wants something, he'll make it happen."

I was so proud of him that I could have burst right there and then.

Mark, the boys and I attended a star-studded event in September of 2014 to watch the other deserving award winners receive their recognition and collect their prizes. Our category was one of the last, and by the time it came around, Oliver was getting tired and a little grumpy.

As the videos were shown for the nominations, I had no idea how the judges would have decided who should win. Harry's story was beautifully explained with some lovely footage of him playing the piano and bouncing on the trampoline at our house. But so were the stories of Peter who had CHARGE syndrome, a cluster of conditions affecting his eyes, ears, heart and growth, and Abbie who had raised over £3,000 by having her hair cut to donate for wigs for other cancer sufferers. All incredible stories, so we were stunned to realise that Harry had won.

Oliver came onto the stage with his brother and me as Harry was presented with an enormous framed certificate, a silver-plated plaque and an envelope full of vouchers for trips and experiences. There was rapturous applause, and while Harry was giggling at the commotion around him, I could see that Oliver was struggling. My tired boy must have felt like Harry had trumped him yet again in the attention stakes, and eventually he had a monumental meltdown. There were tears and tantrums at the dinner table as people came to congratulate Harry, so rather than wait for the rest of the awards to be announced, we decided to leave early.

By the time we got to the car, Oliver was screaming and sobbing hysterically, and I wasn't helping. With a few hundred pairs of eyes on us in the event, I had smiled but hissed at him to calm down, embarrassed and furious at his outburst. Couldn't he see that Harry might have an award, but he had a life his brother would never enjoy? I wanted Oliver to be proud of his brother, but what eight-year-old can do that?

My expectations were ridiculous and unfair. Oliver was simply a boy who was jealous of the huge amount of attention his brother received, tired not only of that long day, but a life that he felt he got the raw end of.

Once I had calmed Oliver I was able to remind him that he too had an award, a picture in the newspaper and an army of loving fans and supporters. I told him about all the things that he would have in the future to look forward to, and back on: travel, jobs, houses, girlfriends. Harry probably wouldn't have those things, so an award now was just a little way of recognising that and making a memory for him. I told Oliver that we loved him very much, and that while his trophy was for him alone to enjoy, he would be taking part in the many free activities that Harry had received.

I cuddled him and I reassured him. Yes, I should have done that at the beginning, but I'm not a perfect person, so on what planet was I ever going to be a perfect mother? Merely one trying her best to do the right thing when she can and learn from her mistakes.

Oliver thought about what I had said and replied, "I'll take him with me when I go on holidays, Mummy. I'll always take care of Haz." And my heart was crushed and burst with pride at the same time. I kissed my boy and reminded him that he was the greatest thing I had ever done.

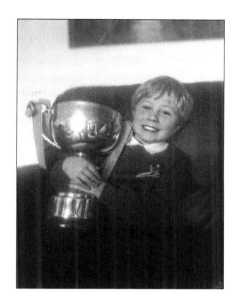

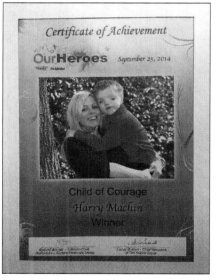

Certificate of Achievement

OurHeroes   September 25, 2014

Child of Courage

Harry Machin

Winner

Planning for the Future

I decided to set up an email account for Oliver, one that I could give to him as an adult so he could read the moments and see pictures I treasured between us. I loved writing to the man he had yet to become.

One evening, Oliver challenged me to describe how much I loved him better than my usual response of "More than the universe". I told him, and then I emailed him my reply.

I love you more than the number of tears you will ever cry, more than the number of times your heart will ever beat, more than the number of lips you will ever kiss. I love you more than all of the beautiful sunrises or sunsets you'll ever see, and more than all of the stars that you will count. I love you more than anything before you or anything since. I love you more than I love myself.

I think he liked that reply, and I loved having a way to record it to remind him in the future when he looks back on a childhood full of challenges. I would highly recommend all parents do this for the siblings of their unique children. It will be my gift at the right time for Oliver. A lifetime of love for him to treasure.

*****

Once I had settled into our new home, I felt it was time to do the grown-up thing and make a will. My sister Emily featured heavily (particularly when it came to arranging the funeral – no black allowed; great music, please), maybe on account of the fact that she's 10 years younger than me and will hopefully still have plenty of life left in her when there is none left in me.

While making my will, I was asked, "Who will be responsible for the care of Harry once you and Mark both die?" and there it was. The question that haunts my dreams and plagues many of my waking moments. Who will be there for my eternal boy when I am gone? The assumption would be Oliver, but I feel that he should be allowed to make that decision for himself later on. Will he even be around to care for Harry? Will life take him exploring and settling elsewhere? Part of me hopes so, part of me hopes not.

And what about Harry? Will he prefer to live in his own specialist accommodation? Will he ever have the mental maturity to understand and decide? I know none of the answers, and so I left that part blank and added it to the ever-growing mental list of things to think about in the future.

249

Harry's Ways

Harry's speech was coming on well. He physically doesn't have the capacity to make some sounds, but he rambles on in his own way, sometimes understandable, often not. But the moments that he can make himself understood are amazing.

When I picked something up of Oliver's, he would tell me, "Dat O-yee-bers," and when I showed him his reflection in the mirror on a school day, he would say, "Ve-yee smart". His negotiation skills were also developing, with his biscuit demands going from "Ten discuits" to "Five discuits" to "Fee discuits" before he grabbed a bowl and waited like Oliver Twist for more gruel.

Often he said single words or a couple to make a short sentence, but one day, as I approached him playing in the yard at his after school club, I heard him shout, "Dare's Mummy. She comiiiiing. She 'ere! Dare's Mummy." I melted in the same way I would have done if he'd been two and saying it. Except, he wasn't two, he was nine, and I was hearing his excitement for the first time in full sentences. I hoped with all of my heart that something was being unlocked within him and his speech would continue to flow and develop. But special needs life isn't like that, and so we would have moments of conversational inspiration then random or unrecognisable words for the weeks that followed.

Although even those have been amusing at times. Like when he picked up the word 'annoying' from Oliver. I collected Harry from school one day after a call to say that he wasn't well and told him that we were going to the doctor. By now Mark and I had created a rod for our own backs after treating Harry to toys for his operations and hospital visits in a bid to get him over his hospital phobia.

"Doctors and den Toys R Us," he said, to which I replied, "No, not today."

He then mumbled, "'nnoying!" with a passion under his breath. I nearly crashed the car, I laughed so hard.

Although his speech was coming on well, nights were still horrendous. As he was a child obsessed with technology, I took his iPad off him before bedtime and we had cuddles and calm for an hour. Yet he fought sleep and would be awake until 11pm some nights, only to have a short power nap and be awake for the day from 2am, banging on his door for my attention. I would sit on his floor with him for a while, but after either a long stint of numb bum or several attempts to leave him to settle only to be yelled at to return, I would climb into his single bed with him, top to toe. There, I would be removing his toes from various orifices and having my legs repositioned to where Harry wanted them in relation to him.

Then, just as I thought he was settling, he would clamber on top of me and turn his head to the right, staring me straight in the face with his one eye to check if I was awake or not. Of course, I pretended not to be, which sometimes worked but often didn't. Harry would bounce on the bed, grab my hand to pull back my fingers or lie at my side to poke and prod my face. He would eventually settle around 5.30am just in time for Oliver to wake at 6.30am, and we would all get up to start our day at school – my boys to learn and me to try to teach.

After one such night, Oliver asked for the 500th time whether we could have a dog. He gave me an extensive list of reasons why a dog would be a great asset to our family, but I was exhausted and barely able to look after the three of us. I explained that on days where I needed to catch up on the sleep I had been denied the previous night, I would feel incredibly guilty for not walking a dog.

Oliver, after being quiet for a moment, hit me with, "I wish my brother wasn't disabled."

On this occasion, I wanted to agree, but I just said, "I know, but it would be boring if we were all the same."

Oliver, as sharp as anything, replied, "OK, he could still have his 'ways', but he wouldn't make you so tired and sad. Mummy, if Harry had come out like me, I think he would have liked *Transformers*. I think he'd have liked Bumblebee and I could be Optimus and we would play together and Harry would sleep like me."

He smiled at me as if it were a possibility, and I smiled back despite the most enormous sob trapped in my throat.

"That would be awesome. We'll have to show him Bumblebee and see if he likes him." But I knew that however Harry reacted to a *Transformers* toy, it would never equal the picture Oliver had just painted. I waved Oliver goodbye, got into my car and sobbed till my tired eyes stung.

Nan, my Hero

We take so much of life for granted. We know that day will follow night and we expect everything and everyone to continue forever.

We all believed this to be true for Nan. At 93 years old she was still visiting my house most days to potter about, wash dishes and generally clean up when I wasn't home (my nan was a cleaning machine) and have some company on the days when I wasn't teaching. I would often stop at my house after teaching to pick her up before collecting the boys from the school club, and we would either take her home on dark nights or wave to her from the landing window on lighter nights as she waited for her 7A bus.

Nanna Mo. She had been there for me as a baby, and the same for my boys. I have so many photographs of feeding and bath times with the boys as babies; tea parties that she had with Oliver under tables; sandwiches on park benches as we walked in the hope of tiring out Harry; visits to the park; days when she sat on the sofa watching all manner of mind-numbing children's TV; birthday parties; concerts. She never missed a day.

In February of 2014 she was taken into hospital with a water infection. My nan, who needed to be out and about, who never stayed in or sat doing nothing, was now in a hospital bed, and her 93 years caught up with her. She had a fall in hospital one evening, and as the one who lived closest, I went to her straight away and accompanied her to A&E.

We chatted and laughed, and in her loud voice, she said, "I think that driver's got his eye on you, Char!" making me feel quite embarrassed. She had a wicked sense of humour at times, and even being called out of bed in the middle of the night was worth it to spend a couple of hours in her company. I didn't just love my nan, I adored and worshipped the very ground she walked on.

After the fall, she deteriorated quickly. She had had cancer about 15 years earlier and it had returned more recently. We knew that her body could only take so much, so we visited daily, watching her and eating her up with our eyes, knowing that we wouldn't have her for much longer.

I took the boys to start with, but soon she didn't look well enough, and their energy tired rather than rejuvenated her, so their visits stopped. But towards the end of March, I was spending as much time as I could at the hospital.

Chatting to me one afternoon, she said from nowhere, "When I'm gone, I'll be able to see the boys every day." My throat closed and I asked her not to talk like that, but she continued as her paper-thin hands held my own and she looked at me with a moment of clarity and a smile.

"I'll always be with you, you know. I'll try to help you as best I can and I'll see you and the boys every day."

"Promise?" was all I could manage, and she promised.

I sat with her daughters for three days solid at the end of March. As I left her quiet and unresponsive figure, I told her that I understood she had to go and that I loved her so very much.

Before I had reached the car park, her condition had deteriorated, and within the hour she was gone. Mum thinks she waited for me to leave. I was bathing the boys at the same time as she left us here on this earth. I can't imagine she would have had it any other way.

Oliver was devastated and still cries about her three years on. I have no idea if some part of Harry felt her loss, and it only added to my sadness that he was totally unaware of the hole that had appeared in our lives and how intensely he had been loved by my hero.

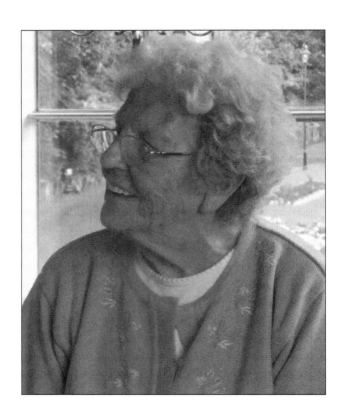

A Holiday and an Eye

Despite feeling exhausted and low from the loss of Nan, I knew that she would want me to be a strong mum for my boys, and so I decided, after much consideration, to take them on our first holiday abroad as a trio. We visited Lanzarote. Although I was worried about the change of location and routine for Harry, we had a fantastic week – mainly thanks to the toys I took which kept him happy when all else failed!

There was absolutely no way that Harry was getting into the chilly pool in October, and as I was unable to leave him unattended, Oliver was left to swim alone a lot of the time. This annoyed rather than upset him, but being the chameleon that he is, he soon adapted and played either with other children or in front of us. When he did the latter, I could dangle my feet in while holding Harry on my knees so that he didn't scream as if he were being murdered every time any water touched him.

These were the times when I wondered at which point Oliver would begin to resent Harry; to feel more than annoyance that Harry's needs and the adaptations we had to make to accommodate them were too unfair on a sibling who wanted to enjoy his life without constraints. But it appeared the holiday wasn't that point and we all had a great week, despite the fact that our room had no air conditioning so I had to leave the door open slightly. I slept with one eye open, too, fearing that Harry would want to explore, or a single mum would make a great target for unwanted visitors. I slept on the crack where the boys' single beds met, and in between checking that they were safe through the night and slipping down into the gap, I felt incredibly proud of myself for managing the break.

*****

When we got home, we were greeted by a letter inviting us to Liverpool eye hospital. Harry's first prosthesis was ready and we would be losing the bright green lump at last.

Andrew came with me as Mark was unable to have the time off work. On the way there, we worried about how Harry would react to having the eye put in, whether he would even notice, and how I would feel on seeing the transformation.

We need not have worried. Although he was anxious at first, we calmed him in the hospital chair and I explained what would be happening. The green mould had been left at home, so all Harry had was the fleshy exposed socket waiting patiently for its new addition.

Unlike the early days, I didn't really think now about the amount of time it was taking for us to create what nature would have done in a matter of days. Those worries were pointless, so I focused on each new stage that was coming with excitement and a little apprehension. The face I loved was changing again, and each time, it took my breath away in a wondrous and emotional way.

The prosthesis was incredible. Where I had expected a round ball-like object, the eye was shaped more like a guitar plectrum with the wider side at the bridge of Harry's nose and the tapered end towards the outer corner of his eye. The detail was outstanding and the likeness to his own eye was amazing: a perfect pupil surrounded by delicate flecks of pale blue and light grey which reached out to a darker edge around the iris.

Harry was relatively calm as the prosthetic worker pushed the eye into his socket. And then, just like that, my boy had two eyes. At his birth, in describing Harry's appearance, Dr Mona had swept his hand across the left side of his face, erasing all the features that were there and leaving only confusion, emptiness and a barren landscape. Now, we were seeing the results of years of operations, disappointments, setbacks and victories come to bloom and I wanted to cry. Every success for Harry felt to me like another layer of armour, another step closer to ensuring that he would be OK. It was one step closer to him having the chance to be accepted because of his merits rather than despite his differences. I can't describe the emotional, physical and mental impact of decisions and days like those. Knowing we had made the right choice when it so easily could have been the wrong one. My boy looked amazing, and his smile at his own reflection felt like a lottery win.

*****

We do have some fun with that eye! I can't count the number of days I have jumped in the car to drive off with the boys, only to realise I've left the eye in water beside the kettle. One day Harry came home from school without his eye, only for it to be found the next day skidding around on the floor of his school bus. It was the first time I could say that my child had a wandering eye.

Then there was the day we supported the When You Wish charity and Harry's eye spontaneously fell out and nearly gave one of the office staff at the company a heart attack. She clutched my arm and, horrified, said, "His eye just fell out!" I laughed so much.

But my favourite eye story has to be the day I got a call from school to tell me it was coming out. I was at the butcher's counter, waiting for the assistant to bag up my meat, so I simply explained that the teacher should press on the inside of the eye next to the bridge of Harry's nose and it would pop straight out. The poor woman serving me literally stood with her mouth open, staring at me until I explained – through giggles. I wasn't laughing when I got home and realised she'd forgotten to pack my mince, but it was funny at the time.

My other favourite Harry giggle is the evening that he sat in the bath as I washed his hair and sang to him. The other three children were downstairs, bickering over something or nothing. They were loud and constant, and I looked at Harry's gorgeous little face and thought how blessed I was to have this placid, quiet soul. As if he knew, he looked up at me, smiled, melted my heart and then shit in the bath. My squeals had him laughing hysterically, and me laughing for years later.

If I have learned anything on this journey, it's to laugh as often as possible. Yes, there will be days that you'll cry, but try to find the humour where you can. It makes for better memories to look back on through the tough times.

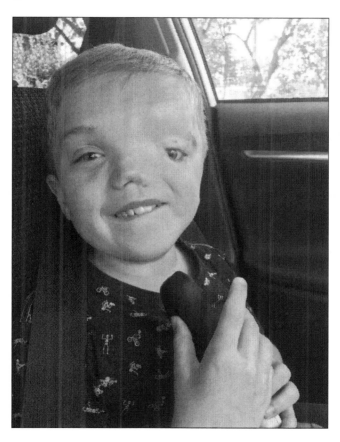

The End of an Era

I was very grateful to be able to take Harry on his appointments, but whereas I had hoped that working part-time would give me some work-life balance, I found that I was still working at home on the days when I wasn't teaching. The stress, as my head teacher had predicted, of sharing a class but feeling the full responsibility of their progress was beginning to take its toll.

That and too many years of sleepless nights, plus more worry in the past nine years than many feel in a lifetime, culminated in me having a horrendous headache at school one Monday afternoon, quickly followed by the loss of vision in one eye. My head teacher sent me home (yes, I drove, and no, I shouldn't have), and by the time I was seen by my local doctor, I was struggling to think through a cloud of fog and my speech was slurring.

I was sent immediately with Mum to A&E with a suspected mini stroke. The *only* thought in my head was for my boys. There was no way on earth that I could be having a stroke when they needed me so much; I still had to keep them safe and help them through their lives. My heart was banging against my chest and my head was swimming.

After countless blood tests, ECG scans and half an aspirin, I was discharged and told to return to the stroke clinic three days later. The doctors were fairly certain that I hadn't had a stroke, but they wanted the cardiologists to take a look at my notes. What they did note was that my blood pressure was so high that they wanted me to rest completely.

My own doctor suggested I take a couple of weeks off work. After one week I felt too guilty being away and returned early, only to be told that my books hadn't been marked up to standard according to a local authority inspection while I had been away. I came home and cried. I loved teaching and the school I taught at, but it was clear that the expectations, pressures and ever changing goalposts of education, coupled with my own sleep-deprived, stressful lifestyle, were making me ill. However, I had no idea what else I could do that would give me the flexibility I needed around my boys and the income I needed as a single parent, and I begged the universe for a way out.

In December 2014 I was approached by a friend of my mum who asked if I would be open to taking a look at a new business opportunity. I went with a weary heart and an open mind, and was introduced to the industry of network marketing. I heard how one unhappy teacher had replaced her income, and dared to dream that I could do the same.

I joined immediately, and 19 weeks later I was matching my income so I resigned from teaching. As I finish my book at long last, I am still a network marketer, and ever grateful for the time that I have with my boys every single day.

The Mischief Maker

Moments when hope shines into your life like sunrays on a cloudy day are priceless. One such moment found me frozen to the spot in the doorway to my lounge as I watched Harry pushing some VTech toy cars along a short track he had put together himself.

"Dis way, Harry," he said.

My boy, who had only ever been interested in cause and effect VTech toys, or watching clips of people making remote controls on YouTube, was finally using his imagination. A world that I'd had no proof existed took my breath away when I saw it for myself. Maybe there's a lesson right there to trust that our unique children simply choose to drip feed us with their brilliance when the time is right for them, and we should never doubt its existence. If we can believe in Santa and help others do the same, then we can trust in the magic within our own children, and in ourselves.

Inside every innocent looking child, though, is a crafty mischief maker waiting to spy their chance. When I have my boys with me, my showers are only short and sweet, but by the time I got out one day, I could smell something acrid and strong.

Dashing downstairs with only a towel around me, I ran into the kitchen as Harry raced out, saying, "Uh oh." Thick black smoke was billowing out the back of the microwave, and as I pulled the door open, I could see why. Two of my best lipsticks, some cutlery and a few plastic items, which had now melted to the glass plate, were looking very sorry for themselves. In the oven, meanwhile, a main course of polo mints and two of Oliver's toys were baking beautifully at 200 degrees. I threw the back door open as quickly as I could, but the smell of burnt plastic clung to the curtains for days and I had to throw my towel away.

My local fire station offered a free service to fit fire alarms, and of course, I hadn't taken advantage of this. Now, I realised that I needed to, and a fitter came out to my house within the week. They asked some great questions on discovering that Harry had autism and said that it would be noted on the system. They explained that in an emergency, the vehicle would approach the house with just lights and no sirens for fear of distressing the child, but I explained that the loud wailing noise of a siren, coupled with the commotion, would probably delight and excite Harry so much that he'd turn into a juvenile arsonist and the fire brigade would be sick of seeing us.

Just lights it is, then!

I couldn't help but laugh at Harry as his personality developed. I was always keen to encourage him to use his voice to express choices, and I started with food. Initially I would show him his options and make him repeat his choice to me several times, but in no time at all, I could say, "Harry, toast today. Do you want jam or honey?" Although I might have to repeat myself a few times, eventually he would choose and I would feel triumphant in helping him have what *he* wanted and not what I decided for him.

One weekend, I took my boys out for lunch. Oliver, like his foodie mother, had decided in no time what he wanted. Harry, meanwhile, was proving slightly trickier.

"Harry, would you like sausage or steak?"

"Sausage or steak."

"No, does Harry want sausage or steak?"

"Sausage or steak."

"No, Harry. Sausage. Or steak."

"Steak."

"Steak?"

"Steak."

"Great. Do you want chips or mash?"

"Chips or mash."

"No, Harry. Do you want chips? Or mash?"

"Chips! Chips!"

"Chips?"

"Chips."

I felt delighted that he had chosen his own food, and when the waitress came to take our order, I proudly turned to Harry.

"Harry, what would you like?"

"Sausage."

I swear he did it on purpose, but he made me roar with laughter and deflate in frustration at the same time.

A Painful Recovery

Just as we relaxed back into the normality of a life that is anything but normal, we had a reminder that disruption is only ever around the corner. In March of 2016, Harry went back to Alder Hey to have his palate stretched. This, compared to many of his other procedures, was relatively straightforward, and at only two-and-a-half hours, quite short, too, but I was more nervous than usual.

The consultant had, as ever, been totally honest and told us that there were no guarantees that this would help Harry's speech at all, but it was worth a try. If the soft palate muscle could reach the back of his throat, then his hard consonant sounds would be much clearer, giving him a better chance of being understood without someone fluent in his dialect being there to translate. However, I feared that the surgery would make him anxious and we would lose the bit of speech that he did have as he became reliant on hand leading and pointing again. This in turn would result in him feeling frustrated and upset. As ever, all we had was hope that it would help him at best and make no difference at worst.

After the operation, the surgeon informed us that there was far more muscle wastage than he had expected, and while he had gone ahead and performed the operation, he wasn't confident that it would help. I hoped and prayed that Harry would recover quickly and not regress at all.

He stayed in the high dependency unit at Alder Hey for two nights. Due to the nature of the ward, parents didn't usually stay, but I couldn't leave him and slept at his bedside in an upright plastic visitors' chair with my hands through the side rail of his bed so he knew I was there. Looking around that ward, I really appreciated how fortunate we are. It's flippant to say that there's always someone who's got it worse than you, and although it's most definitely true, I don't think anyone actually appreciates the fact until they are staring it in the face.

The girl in the bed next to Harry was paralysed from her neck down and only able to communicate through grunting sounds. An infant had more wires attached to him than I've ever seen. In the middle of the night, another girl crashed and the resuscitation team raced in to save her. And all the time, my boy slept and I stroked his hand and thanked my lucky stars that our life wasn't that traumatic; that our struggles weren't that intense; that our hope wasn't stretched quite that far.

*****

For 24 hours, Harry couldn't even swallow his own saliva. He woke with his mouth caked in congealed blood, and he was silent. No requests for 'discuits', remotes or VTech toys. No chattering away. Just grimaces and the odd groan. I tried to explain to him what had happened and that he would be better soon, but I wasn't sure how much of it he had understood.

I brought him home after two days and fed him only yoghurts and sips of juice. It was painful to watch, and it must have been excruciating for Harry. Within a week, my already petit boy was losing weight and his face felt tiny as I cupped it in my hands. No fleshy cheeks to pinch and snuggle into, just bone and pain.

As he began to talk again, he must have realised that something was physically different and he tried, hundreds of times a day, to put his fingers down his throat. Each time we had to stop him for fear of infection, and over the next few weeks he became obsessed with gaining permission to swallow. He would take a mouthful of juice and hold it for minutes on end. He would hesitate in picking up his food and have to be encouraged to chew and swallow, often spitting it out instead. At times he would put his whole hand into his mouth, and when that didn't ease his discomfort, he lashed out, usually hurting himself. On one occasion, as he sat at my side with a fork loaded and ready for the next battle, he stabbed it into the back of his tongue and made his mouth fill with blood. It was relentless and draining for everyone.

I regretted allowing the operation as I watched my boy waste away and turn against himself, but we persevered, knowing there was no other option. I took him to the doctor, to the dentist, and finally requested another appointment with the surgeon. Everyone reported that they were pleased with his progress and had no idea where the behaviour came from.

It lasted for months, and then, as quickly as it had begun, it was gone. My boy ate normally again and his self-harming stopped. He put on weight, and I no longer wanted to cry, watching my walking bag of bones climb into the bath. He was on the mend, and my chatty boy returned.

Pokémon No!

I don't think Harry's recovery was helped by the timing of him getting ready to leave Springfield for high school. Mark and I had visited two schools that we were interested in, the first being across the driveway from his current school and the second being 12 miles away in Newcastle-under-Lyme. After visiting them both, we knew that Harry would feel more settled and at home in the second school where music played from classrooms and corridors were lined with class-made displays of colour and creativity. In the same way that you view several houses until you find the home that feels right, Blackfriars felt right for us, and we knew we wanted Harry to go there from Year Seven onwards.

I explained to Harry that big school was coming, but I think he already knew that change was afoot and he was struggling to cope. His tantrums, previously aimed at himself, now turned to hitting others – Oliver, Harrison, me and his peers. He was volatile and unpredictable for the first time in his life, coupled with a superhuman strength and lack of self-control, and I was worried. Visits out were proving even more challenging than before.

At the height of the Pokémon Go craze, I took Harry and Oliver, who was desperate for a Dragnonite (don't ask!), around a local mere to capture the elusive creature. Harry was having none of it. He threw himself to the floor, screaming like he was having his limbs removed, and kicked me as I tried to get close. Approaching from another angle, I was able to slip my arms under his armpits and pull him up onto his feet, only for him to throw himself back down again as he wriggled free, smacked himself in the head and screeched.

The other visitors to the mere were watching on in fascination or horror. I didn't know which. Some pointed, some whispered behind their hands (by the way, that doesn't make you invisible), and one lady came over to offer her assistance as a special needs practitioner. On one hand I was genuinely touched, yet at the same time I was embarrassed that a stranger should have to intervene, and I was furious at Harry for creating a sideshow and spoiling Oliver's time yet again.

Oliver himself panicked and repeatedly said, "It's OK, Mum, we can go. We can go. It doesn't matter," but I knew that it did matter to him and I was determined that Harry would walk around that mere.

Eventually I got him to his feet, and the three of us 'walked' – sometimes I dragged, sometimes carried, sometimes skipped with Harry. Oliver excitedly told me the facts and figures of his latest obsession, and though I struggled to hear a word of it over Harry's shouts and protests, I smiled and nodded anyway.

A New School

I attended some transition sessions with Harry at the new school, terrified that the staff wouldn't understand him and concerned that I'd have no way of knowing whether he was enjoying it or not. The staff were fantastic, and Harry's new TA reassured me that she'd felt exactly the same when her boys went to high school. She promised she'd take him under her wing, and I believed her.

I stayed with him for the first session and was astounded at the size of some of the children sharing his playground. Many of them were taller than me (not that that's difficult as I'm the height of a hobbit), and I wanted to scoop him up and take him home. At break time, one of the pupils approached us to tell us that Harry's face was freaking him out. I explained why he looked different and that he could only see out of one eye. The boy's face lit up as he said that he too could only see out of one eye.

"I'll look after him," he said, and I smiled at this gentle giant, taller than me but developmentally younger than I would have ever guessed.

I did like that Harry's class teacher was firm, like Lisa had been. He needed that, and I could sense that he would get clear boundaries with a sprinkling of cuddles. When I was ever so politely encouraged to bugger off and leave them to it 30 minutes into the second session, my heart was in my mouth, but I felt a little easier than I had before. I took photographs of the staff home with me, and chatted to Harry often about the new faces, both staff and pupils, that he would see from September.

But Harry struggled to cope with the change. His sleeping was worse than ever, his aggression was getting worse, too, and unbeknown to me, my boy was hatching a plan which would unravel me for months to come.

The Great Escape

One Thursday in the school holidays, as Oliver and I snuggled together watching a film, there was a knock at the door. Oliver came with me to answer it as his insecurities meant that an unexpected knock made him nervous, and we were greeted by the friendly Asian guy from the petrol station across the road.

"Your son," he said. I was confused. Oliver was with me, and Harry was upstairs, playing with the Thomas the Tank Engine in his bedroom.

"Little. Your son," the guy continued.

"Yes? He's upstairs."

"No, he's over there."

The man motioned across the busy road in front of my house with its constant stream of traffic and my heart jumped out of my chest. Without thinking, I dashed out of my driveway and across the road to the garage.

Bursting in, I found Harry squealing loudly with utter delight, bouncing up and down and flapping his arms as if he were trying to take flight. It took me a second to realise that he was totally naked behind the frantic customer who was trying to cover him with her fleece held out like a matador's cape. His arms weren't the only thing flapping, and Harry was loving it!

I picked him up quickly and threw him onto my hip. A customer at the garage informed me that I couldn't leave as the police were on their way, but I barged my way past him to return home with Harry laughing hysterically.

I had been gone for two minutes at the most and the petrol station was in clear view for Oliver, but me dashing away unexpectedly had him in a hysterical meltdown. He was screaming down the phone and sobbing uncontrollably.

I took the phone off him to find that he'd understandably called Mark. Now as good as Mark is, I didn't want him judging me as a bad parent. I explained that I was sorting everything, then in temper threw Oliver's phone back at him and it smashed, leaving him even more upset.

Meanwhile, Harry was clambering onto the trampoline to continue his naked bouncing, flapping and squealing as the police pulled up at the house. I grabbed his legs and dressed him from the pile of clothes he had stripped off before his great escape. I was glad he was safe, angry that he had run off and mortified that the police were at my door. Although I totally understood why. The poor guy in the petrol station must have wondered what on earth was going on.

The police were understanding and patient as I calmed Oliver, quietened Harry from his relentless laughter, and tried to steady my own nerves. I explained that Oliver and I had been watching a film and that Harry must have crept downstairs, out of the patio door (which he'd silently closed behind him), around the side of the house and through the gate before stripping off by the trampoline and streaking across to the garage. The police were stunned that he hadn't been hit by a car, and I was tormented for days after with the 'what if?' scenarios.

I had no idea why he went across the road, but I assured the police that it would not be happening again. They could see that it wasn't a safeguarding issue, and that Harry was well looked after, not an escapee from some special needs child trafficking racket. They said they would see if Social Care could get in touch and offer support. I explained that I would willingly accept any help available, and the police left us all to recover from what was rapidly feeling like the impact of a collision.

Not since Harry's escape as an infant had I felt so scared, sick, relieved and drained. Oliver was a mess. I hugged him to me and explained that I had left him in the house only for a few minutes while I brought Harry back and that I was always returning, but that fear of being abandoned triggered his anxieties again. For months afterwards he needed to know the room I was in and I had to dictate all of my movements with a running commentary.

Harry was relentless. We padlocked the gate closed as we waited to have a 6ft fence erected across the garden, but still he tried to escape. I caught him trying to scale the short picket fence between us and the neighbours the day after his garage escapade and eventually walked him across the road myself to see what the attraction was. There was nothing, and touch wood, Harry hasn't tried to get across the road again since.

They are frustratingly, grey hair generating, mysterious creatures, these unique children of ours!

The Young Carer

The boys' birthday in June was, for the first time, celebrated twice. Oliver had a surprise trip in a stretch Hummer with a birthday playlist, compiled by me, blaring as he and 13 of his friends were taken out for lunch. Harry enjoyed the energetic chaos of the day, but as his imaginative play had grown into an obsession with Thomas the Tank Engine, we decided to treat him to a day at Thomas Land as his birthday celebration.

He was excited to be there, but clearly overwhelmed at times. When Andrew and I saw him with his arm around Oliver on one of the rides, we were laughing at first, until we realised that Harry had Oliver in a headlock and was punching him in the head. I couldn't get to them to intervene so we were helpless, waiting until the ride had finished, at which point Oliver cried and shouted repeatedly that he hated Harry and wished he could punch him back. Harry just laughed, which only made matters worse.

Moments later, Oliver was in tears again, feeling awful for saying that he hated his brother but full of resentment for the moments that Harry spoiled. Of everyone, it was Oliver who bore the brunt of Harry's frustration most. Saying that it was because Harry loved him the most did little to help, and not for the first time, Oliver wished for a normal brother. My heart sank (as my fingers were bent backwards for the fiftieth time). The protector had become the prey and all I could do was hope that this latest phase passed soon.

Someone from Social Care visited and decided that we were a 'family in crisis'. Harry was referred for psychological support and Oliver was referred to the Young Carers' Association. I feared that he wouldn't attend as he had refused the same help some years earlier, but this time he was ready for the break and actually enjoyed the recognition that he was a young carer and that Harry wasn't the only one having challenges at home. It gave a context to his battles with and on behalf of Harry, and made him feel important and not just different.

When the Young Carers' Association visited Oliver's school and asked if there were any young carers there, he proudly raised his hand. He saw it as a badge of honour, a positive recognition for his struggles that many of the pupils around him had no idea about until then. For the first time, Oliver felt it was good to be different, and I was thrilled as he enjoyed the evening and weekend activities that the Young Carers' Association provided.

A Military Operation

We made the best of the summer holidays and prayed that Harry's temper and mood would calm again once he was settling in at school, but before September could come, we had one more curve ball to work with.

Harry had his regular eye check and it was discovered that the sight in his only eye had deteriorated slightly and he needed glasses. That in itself wasn't too traumatic, but he's only got one ear and so the left arm of his glasses was missing a ledge. A sports band was attached to the arms of the glasses, and my boy, as cute as a button, froze completely before tilting his head to stop them sliding off, moving like he had the world's stiffest neck.

As much as he smiled at his reflection, he insisted they were taken "Off! Off!" And so as well as the tantrums, the fights and the security watch of Harry Houdini, over the summer we also had five-minute intervals of, "Glasses on. Wait for the beep," until the oven timer went off. I often think I need one of those signs that says *You don't have to be mad to live here, but it helps.*

Mark and his partner Rachel decided to take the boys abroad in the August of 2016. Mark hadn't taken

Harry away the previous year as he had felt that Oliver wasn't getting the quality time and experience that he deserved with Harry there. While I totally got that, I found it hard to consider a holiday without him.

They went to Portugal for a week, and I waited anxiously for reports of how he was getting on because Andrew and I were taking the four children for our first foreign holiday together to Ibiza in the October.

Portugal was a disaster. Harry had screamed the plane down on the flight out and been removed first when it landed because he was so distressed (as were the rest of the passengers, from all accounts). This unfortunately set the tone for the rest of the week. The weather was hot, Harry wasn't sleeping well, and the Wi-Fi was hit and miss, so more than once he launched his iPad across the pool side in frustration, knocking other holidaymakers' drinks flying. If Mark went off for an hour with Oliver, he would return to find Rachel exhausted and helpless to calm Harry. One night, Mark woke up to hear the clunk of the hotel door and discovered Harry Houdini doing a midnight flit. Nights after that were spent barricaded in the hotel room.

On his return, Mark strongly advised that I leave Harry with him while the other children enjoyed the break, but I just couldn't do it. I knew I was risking the smooth running of our first family holiday abroad and could potentially be spoiling it for the others, but without Harry we weren't a family, and so 'Operation Ibiza' was born.

We hired a portable Spanish Wi-Fi router so that we had access to technology at all times; I bought five cheap toys and wrapped them for a grand reveal every other day; Lisa (who was still in touch with us and willing to help) made and laminated some cards showing all the activities we would be doing – including the standard eating, drinking, iPad cards – and I made a 'now and next' board with Velcro. I also laminated 10 pictures of the hotel, five pictures of gifts and one picture of Mark and Harry so that he could tear them off the Velcro daily and have a visual countdown. We took a bag full of Thomas track and trains and a few of the remote controls that he was still obsessed with.

It was like a military operation, but it was all worth it. The holiday was an incredible success, and other than two episodes where Harry got distressed (Andrew actually has a scar where Harry took a chunk out of his back with his nails), it was fantastic and I felt proud of us all. I took so much for granted before Harry, and appreciate every small victory and extraordinary ordinary moment now.

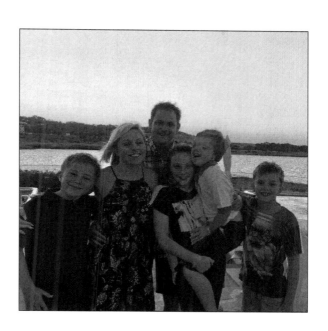

New Experiences

Back at home, Harry was loving his new school in no time. Although I was terrified to be told that he would be going on his first full week residential holiday just three weeks into the term, I hoped that this would be the time for the staff and pupils to really get to know each other and I reluctantly agreed. My plan was to travel to the Lake District for a midweek overnight stay and bring Harry home if he wasn't settling.

However, the universe has a funny way of working things out. A free holiday to Greece that I had qualified for with my company was scheduled for the same week. I had no choice but to let Harry go away without me for the very first time. With people who were still getting to know him and without a familiar face or routine to reassure him.

I worried and asked for daily updates, but, as ever, my concerns were unfounded. Not only did Harry have a great five days, but he made a new friend. Billy walked more slowly than most and Harry had held his hand and walked beside him. When Harry struggled to sleep, Billy gave him his teddy, and at the end of the residential, when the children were able to spend their own money, Billy bought a teddy for Harry to take home.

My heart melted to hear that my eternal boy was making friendships, and as scary as it was to let the control go and allow him to enjoy life without me at his side, I knew that it had to happen. Actually, my over-protectiveness sometimes served me much more than it served him. It was time to realise that he would be making an independent life over the next eight years at Blackfriars, and while I was afraid, I was also incredibly proud.

*****

As well as 2016 being the first year Andrew and I had a family holiday abroad, it was also the first Christmas Day we all woke up to together. Harry was as excited as ever to be opening presents (anyone's presents were fair game, as Frankie & Benny's staff, who had to re-wrap 15 empty boxes below their tree, will testify), and Oliver later told me that it had been wonderful to have Benedicta and Harrison to talk and laugh with. I had never even thought of how lonely a Christmas morning must have been for him without a brother to get excited with, but the twinge of sadness lasted only a second as I realised just how lucky I was, watching them all laughing and squealing with excitement.

Benedicta read out the names on the gifts and passed them over. Harry bounced and flapped with super force fuelled by Santa, and all of us, even the non-believer Oliver, felt the magic of being together. I have never felt richer in all of my life than I felt looking at that scene. Of course, I had never imagined me and my boys with anyone other than Mark at Christmas in the beginning, but I felt elated to have this family, this love and this life now.

"Cose ma Eyes!"

January saw discussions with the surgical team about Harry's new ear – or glasses ledge, as I affectionately call it – and we knew that Phase 2 of his reconstruction was beginning. We had been firm in our decision not to allow the use of rib cartilage and skin grafts to fashion a natural ear. Instead, we were opting for a prosthetic copy of his right ear, which would be initially glued and then attached by means of a magnet below the skin. The procedure would be much less invasive, much quicker, and actually give incredible results. It also meant that Harry would be getting a summer and a winter ear as he grew, as apparently, men's ears change colour in the summer. Now if that's not a pub quiz winning fact, I don't know what is!

Harry had been hospital-phobic for years, so as a reward (or perhaps a bribe) for being brave, we would take him to Toys R Us when we got home. One such occasion was when Harry needed to show his penis to the paediatrician, but sat facing away and protesting in his chair until Mark and I exchanged 'the look'.

I said, "Harry, show the doctor your tail, and then Toys R Us."

He was *up*, thrusting his privates at Dr Mona and frantically unzipping his jeans, shouting, "Tail and den Toys R Us," as the doctor laughed and covered his eyes.

However, what often feels like a good idea at the time can come back to bite you with an autistic child who decides that this lovely treat is going into the memory bank. And so, when in January I told Harry we were off to the doctor the next day, he simply grinned at me and cried, "Yeay! Hos-pickle and den Toys R Us." Cut to amused eye rolling on my part and sofa-wrecking bouncing on his.

Similarly, the routine we had created in Ibiza with the gifts every other day was haunting us, too. Harry had sat at the breakfast table and covered both eyes (even the glass one, which I found adorable), and then counted down "Fee-two-one" to his wrapped gift being revealed. From nowhere, a month or so after coming home, he started again, so we gave him the odd remote controls that friends had donated to the 'Mote Cause'.

In no time at all, we had daily doses of "Cose ma eyes. Cose ma eyes. Fee-two-one!" and either deflated Harry when he realised there was no gift or ecstatic Harry to find yet another remote control in front of him. Before long, everyone who knocked on the door was expected to bring a gift. The window cleaner, the FedEx delivery guy, and any friend or family member was subjected to "Cose ma eyes". If a gift didn't appear, Harry would cry, smack himself and lash out. What had begun with great intentions and turned into cute, amusing behaviour was now an obsession which was getting out of hand.

Mark decided to take Oliver skiing in the February half term and I felt that Harry deserved a change of scenery too, so I booked us into a lovely hotel in the Vegas of the North – Blackpool. Don't ever forget your hand sanitiser if you visit. The smell of twopence pieces on my hands for the arcades made me retch!

This was my chance to put "Cose ma eyes" to bed, and so I hid the wrapped remotes in various places around the hotel and asked a couple of different members of staff to hand them over – once at breakfast and once for room service. Harry knew that the remotes were gifts 'from Blackpool' rather than people, so we could say to him later, "No, Harry, the remotes are in Blackpool." I prayed it would work.

He absolutely loved the whole weekend, from the remotes to the bone-shaking ancient rollercoasters which my little adrenaline junkie dragged me on, to the thrill of riding the tram and his first experience of a Jacuzzi. He was desperate to give it a go, but as he wasn't yet 12, I told him I would smuggle him in as long as he used his little voice. I whispered my instructions, but Harry loved the acoustics of the swimming pool, and so as soon as his cute little behind touched the Jacuzzi bubbles, he yelled, "YEEEEAY! BUBBLES! VTECH PHONE AND MOTES AND BUBLES."

Discretion and autism go together like a square peg in a round hole.

Sipping a glass of wine on our final night as a windswept and fresh-air-weary Harry and I awaited room service, I raised a toast and shared it with my incredible Facebook community, who had watched the live broadcasts of Harry's next 'mote' discovery with anticipation, delight and never-ending love, support and encouragement.

Here's to Blackpool, to motes, to rides, to the tram, to my boy laughing his head off, to so many cuddles, to memories! I know everyone thinks I've always got my shit together 24/7, but sometimes, doing things like this with a boy who needs structure and routine, I'm scared. Here's to being brave, to doing it for my boy and with my boy, for the mum he's created, the love I have for him and for all mums of unique children who worry that they can't...until they know that they can.

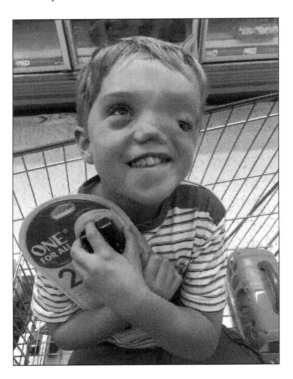

Superpowers

I'm not the woman I was 12 years ago and this is not the life I imagined back then. In many ways it's harder, and in so many ways it's better. In the early days I asked, "Why me?" and "Why him?" Now there's not a day that passes when I don't thank God it was me and I'm so glad he's mine.

Today as I get him dressed for school, at every possible opportunity I kiss or cuddle him. I try this with both of my boys, but pre-teen Oliver is just having none of it! As I dry Harry's face after teeth time, I cup it in my hands and kiss his little lips; as I put his jacket on and zip it up, I nuzzle into his neck to kiss him and he giggles and pushes me away; as I hand him over to his transport chaperone, I touch my head, my heart and then Harry's chest as I say, "I. Love. You." Sometimes he returns the gesture. Most days he just plays with his remotes and wanders off, oblivious to how much I adore the very bones of him.

Then I drop Oliver at school and we have our rock star salute of a screwed up face and tongue out between our first and little fingers as he walks away. He smiles and winks, and I always sit and watch him disappear up the road. My boys. My heartbeat. My world. I am so proud of us all that I could cry.

When my boys were born, I remember sobbing that I couldn't say that Harry had beautiful eyes. 'Beautiful eye' felt wrong. But recently, laughing and bouncing with my sunshine boy, I had a moment where I caught the twinkle in that beautiful eye so full of fun, love and mischief, and it got me thinking. If I could go back 11 years to the broken mother I had just become, I would say this:

You don't have a clue where you are or what's going on, you don't want to be here, and yes, it's shit. It's so unbelievably and catastrophically shit and unfair, but it won't always feel this bad. This dark. You won't always feel this lost. It was not your fault. You did not fail your boy. He will be amazing, and so will you. And that awful hole in your heart that hurts you so much now that you wonder how you'll ever feel anything other than loss will be filled with a love so incredible that you'll thank your lucky stars that Harry came to you (even though you want to punch everyone in the throat who is saying it now).

Don't ever give up on yourself or your boys. The peace you crave now will come. Be strong. Your journey won't always be an easy one, and yes there will be bad days when you question your decisions and doubt yourself, but aren't there in every life?

You are yet to witness the magic of your child and how he will transform you. Be patient. Be kind to yourself. Talk to those closest to you, and please don't feel that you need to be strong for everyone else. Have the pity party you need, just don't live there. You are stronger than you could ever imagine, and an incredible, selfless, fierce warrior mother is already within you. Take one day at a time, and please don't waste precious moments in grief and anger. You will look back one day and regret the bitterness that robbed you of so much joy.

I know you feel like the world has fallen apart now, but know that in time, your boys will create a mosaic masterpiece of the shattered pieces. It's going to be fine. You are going to be fine. Better than fine. I promise.

*****

And so ends our journey so far. We have much still ahead of us. So much is unknown and unpredictable. Sometimes my head buzzes with questions and swims with concerns, but I have to ground myself in the moment and remind myself that worrying doesn't make the answer appear any sooner, so it's better to try my best each and every day. To bring the best of who I am to the table each morning (even if, after a particularly sleep-deprived evening, face down in a bowl of cornflakes is as good as it gets).

I wasn't prepared for any of this. In all of my years of reading books and poems about special needs, *Welcome to Holland* by Emily Perl Kingsley sums it up the best. I took a copy back to the Special Care unit where my boys spent their first six weeks, and I am told that a lot of parents draw comfort from it, so it's my gift to you now. That, and a promise that whatever life throws your way, you can handle it. You were made differently to the others. Like a Marvel Hero, except you're the hero of your own story, and your superpower is a strength beyond words.

Enjoy it all. Be grateful for it all – the torment and pain; the grief and loss; the acceptance and love; the decisions and fears; the relief and the pride; the twists, turns, dead ends and broken satnav on the journey of a special needs family. I have hated it, I have resented it, I have treasured and cherished it, but in the end, I never gave up on it. And if you, like me, are a special needs parent treading the boards for the very first time, good luck. I wouldn't change *Our Altered Life* for a golden pig.

Wishing you every happiness in yours.

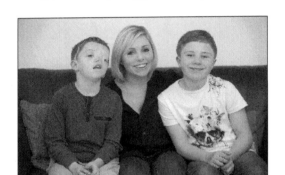

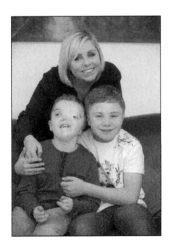

Welcome To Holland

by
Emily Perl Kingsley

I am often asked to describe the experience of raising a child with a disability - to try to help people who have not shared that unique experience to understand it, to imagine how it would feel. It's like this......

When you're going to have a baby, it's like planning a fabulous vacation trip - to Italy. You buy a bunch of guide books and make your wonderful plans. The Coliseum. The Michelangelo David. The gondolas in Venice. You may learn some handy phrases in Italian. It's all very exciting.

After months of eager anticipation, the day finally arrives. You pack your bags and off you go. Several hours later, the plane lands. The flight attendant comes in and says, "Welcome to Holland."

"Holland?!?" you say. "What do you mean Holland?? I signed up for Italy! I'm supposed to be in Italy. All my life I've dreamed of going to Italy."

But there's been a change in the flight plan. They've landed in Holland and there you must stay.

The important thing is that they haven't taken you to a horrible, disgusting, filthy place, full of pestilence, famine and disease. It's just a different place.

So you must go out and buy new guide books. And you must learn a whole new language. And you will meet a whole new group of people you would never have met.

It's just a <u>different</u> place. It's slower-paced than Italy, less flashy than Italy. But after you've been there for a while and you catch your breath, you look around.... and you begin to notice that Holland has windmills....and Holland has tulips. Holland even has Rembrandts.

But everyone you know is busy coming and going from Italy... and they're all bragging about what a wonderful time they had there. And for the rest of your life, you will say "Yes, that's where I was supposed to go. That's what I had planned."

And the pain of that will never, ever, ever, ever go away... because the loss of that dream is a very very significant loss.

But... if you spend your life mourning the fact that you didn't get to Italy, you may never be free to enjoy the very special, the very lovely things ... about Holland.

Mark's View

How did you feel right at the beginning?

I was overjoyed to have two boys! While Charlene was being sewn back together after the C section, I went over to the plastic incubators to meet my little men.

Oliver was perfect, and I remember feeling like I could burst with excitement, but as I walked across the room to where Harry was, the nurse quickly covered half of his face. Then they were both whisked away. I felt a bit uneasy at that point, but we knew they'd be taken to Special Care quickly as they were so premature, so I pushed it to the back of my mind and went back to Charlene.

While she rested on the ward, I called our parents to tell them the news. Everyone was thrilled and asked if I'd seen the boys yet, but I wanted to wait until Charlene was up to it so we could meet them for the first time together. I felt so proud, happy and excited. Nothing beats the feeling of announcing your children's arrival to the world and realising that you're finally a dad!

How did you feel when you were told about Harry?

When I got back to Charlene, we were joined by Dr

Mona who told us the news that we had never expected. Charlene looked stunned and started to cry. I couldn't take it all in. But with Charlene in such a state and still recovering from surgery, I knew I had to be strong. I had to get her through this.

Dr Mona said that both boys were stable but that didn't comfort me much. He hadn't said they were both healthy or doing well, and 'stable' to me didn't necessarily mean that they were OK. I wondered if both of my boys would have problems and what on earth that would mean for us all. It's sad to say that in the space of a few minutes, the happiest day of my life became the saddest.

How did you feel meeting your boys for the first time?

I had mixed emotions, really. On one hand I was amazed to finally see the two little people who had grown within Charlene for the last seven months. We had talked to them, planned and dreamed for them, and to see our little creations was just amazing. But I also felt confused and shocked. I didn't know what to think or feel. I didn't know what to say or expect, so I functioned on autopilot and tried to nod and smile in all the right places. I just knew that I had to stay strong for my new family.

What did you think of Harry's face?

I don't think I really knew what to expect. I noticed straight away that his eye was missing, but I hoped that there would be one underneath the skin that was there instead. I compared the shape of his head to Oliver's and noticed that they weren't quite the same. Harry's jaw did look slightly lopsided, but I just thought that it would look better when he grew a bit more.

His nose was so small that I didn't notice the lack of a nostril at first, and I only realised that he didn't have an ear when the doctor pointed it out to me. It was like I had forgotten everything the doctor had described. Don't forget that the boys were only 3lb 9oz, so as well as everything else, they were also incredibly tiny and wrinkly. To assess so many things in one take was simply mind-blowing.

I know that I wanted some reassurance from the doctor that this could all be 'fixed' and Harry would be looking like his brother in no time. I know that sounds unfair now, but I was in shock and had no idea of the complexity of restructuring Harry's face. I just wanted the babies we had planned for.

I briefly saw the boys on my own first. Although I had wanted to wait for Charlene, she was too upset to see them straight away. I knew she would struggle to take it all in. We had been ridiculously excited about our life with our children. She had been really proud to be carrying twins, and she had looked after herself and the babies so well throughout her pregnancy. She's also one of those people who is never satisfied unless a job is perfect. I worried for her and for myself as I tried to take it all in.

What happened next?

After I met the boys, I called my parents back. I played it down to them because I didn't want to believe it was true. I wanted to carry on as I had been doing a few hours earlier, before everything had changed. Part of me was also scared that they'd think I had failed them; let them down as a son by not giving them two 'perfect' grandchildren. I felt embarrassed and even a bit ashamed right then.

I don't know what I expected them to say, if I'm honest – maybe gasps and exclamations of "Oh my God!", but they were very calm. I remember my dad saying, "It will be OK. Everything will be fine," and his words calmed me.

I found a quiet few minutes to speak with Dr Mona and I remember asking him "Will he ever drive?" Even now I'm amazed at how random that was, but my brain was thinking of all the things that dads do with their sons. They show them how to kick a ball, help them to ride a bike, teach them how to drive a car. That's what I wanted to do with my boys. It's what I had expected would happen in our future. I had a million and one questions, but Dr Mona had no answers for me.

Even now, whenever I see dads with their children, I think, *You don't realise how lucky you are*. It's not that I don't love Harry, but I see the life we could have had. The life we were so confident was ours and suddenly it was gone.

How did you feel when Harry was transferred to Salford?

In the early hours after the boys' birth, when Harry was transferred to Hope Hospital in Salford, I followed the ambulance and went with him. Charlene was with Oliver and I didn't want Harry to be alone.

The SCBU at Salford was bigger, darker and busier than Macclesfield. I sat there for hours with my brain thinking 100 things at 100mph. I don't know what I was thinking about – everything, anything and nothing.

Eventually a nurse suggested that I go and get some rest. It felt like a lifetime since I'd had the call to say that Charlene was going to theatre, and I'd been awake for more than 24 hours. I don't know whether I slept when I got to the car, but suddenly it all hit me. I remember sitting and crying.

How did you cope in those early weeks?

I took some time off work and spent it visiting Harry in Hope Hospital in between morning and late night visits to Charlene and Oliver in Macclesfield. I didn't really see anyone else for the first week and I told no one what had happened. I ignored phone calls and just sent brief texts. It was easier than answering lots of questions, and I used the fact that the boys were premature to explain why they were still in hospital.

I consciously talked about them both the same way. It made them equal in my mind and that helped me at the beginning. I just kept thinking, *If I think they will be fine, then they will be fine.*

My parents had told me everything would be OK on the day the boys were born and it helped then, but as we moved through the week and I was tired from the emotional impact, as well as the 100 mile round trip every day, I didn't want to hear it.

I remember snapping at them and shouting, "Stop saying it! You don't know that everything will be OK. *We* don't know if everything will be OK." I was like a pressure cooker. I didn't want to get upset in front of Charlene as she was struggling to cope anyway. I didn't want to fall apart in front of my parents, and I wasn't talking to anyone else about it. My brothers asked questions and I told them what I knew, but I never got upset with them, even though I wanted to sometimes. I was trying to get on with one day at a time because there was no other option really.

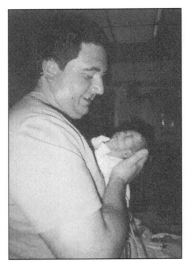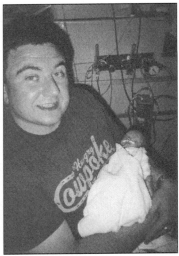

Did you want to know what had caused Harry's condition?

Charlene was convinced she had caused Harry's problems and she thought I would be mad at her, but I honestly never blamed her. I knew she'd had a great, happy, healthy pregnancy and she had looked after herself really well. I did wonder if it was a genetic issue that was out of our control, though – maybe one of hers, maybe one of mine, maybe a rogue combination. I just didn't know.

I remembered being at high school as a young teenager and finding out that one of my friends had an older brother who was disabled. We never talked about him, and only found out that my friend even had a brother by chance. I felt sorry for him and his parents, and for a good few years throughout high school, it really played on my mind that if they could have a disabled child, then maybe I would, too, one day.

Occasionally, in the years since having the boys, I have thought about that. Did I think about it so hard that I made it happen? Did I wish it upon us somehow? Did some part of me as a child already know what I was going to face as a father? Is life mapped out for us already? It makes you wonder.

What about life once the boys came home?

Life was as hard as it is with twins in general, but we had to watch Harry's feeding and sleeping all the time, too, so that put extra pressure on us.

In many ways, the boys were the same. They both fed, slept, cried, etc., and we were generally exhausted from the daytime worries, constant feeds and watching Harry throughout the night, but I was worried about Charlene. She wouldn't go out of the house unless I was with her, and even then she wasn't herself. She loves a project and being organised, so she had spent loads of time while she was pregnant researching the best double buggy for us to use. Some days I wanted to say, "Get a grip and go for a walk", but on the days when we did go out together I was reminded of why it was so hard for her on her own. A double buggy attracts a lot of attention, and more than once we had people coming over to peer into the seats before their faces changed.

"Oh?" they'd say.

"OK!" I'd say and just walk off, pushing the buggy, but I knew it was crushing Charlene.

After a few weeks, she started walking the boys around the local reservoir where it was quiet and she could walk in peace. Then I couldn't keep her in, and she even became a bit obsessed with her lakeside walks, but going out in public was still hard. I suppose, looking back, I didn't always give her enough credit for what she was doing while I was at work. She was dealing with the professionals and the questions and stares, although I think she looked for them sometimes, expecting people to judge us and be mean.

We talked a lot about Harry's medical appointments and the practicalities of having the boys, but I don't think we talked enough about how we were feeling right at the beginning. If I could give any advice to other parents, it would be to talk to each other, even if it means you get upset together. It does help, and now I know that silence can be dangerous in a relationship.

How did you feel about Harry being diagnosed with autism?

Harry's autism diagnosis wasn't a massive shock as his progress was so different to Oliver's, so it didn't affect me as much as it did Charlene. Again, she blamed herself, but I just saw it as something else to deal with. I did know, though, that it would make it harder for him to go to school with Oliver.

I really didn't want him to go to a special school. I wanted him to be 'normal' and still hoped that he would 'get better'. I constantly hoped that he would catch up and have a life like Oliver's, but as time went on, I began to realise that this wouldn't happen. His life would always be different to the one I'd had planned for him.

Do you still feel like that now?

My friend has twin boys. They are the best of friends; they go to school together; they enjoyed their first prom together. That's what I'd been dreaming of for my children, and for a long time I lived in a mixture of denial and hope that Harry would 'outgrow' his problems or be 'fixed' by the doctors so that he could grow into a life that was waiting for him.

Sometimes, yes, I do still feel like that, but not as much. It's hard not to when you see Oliver growing up and going through the typical trials and tribulations of high school. I don't really get upset that Harry's life is different to Oliver's now, but I do wonder what he'll be able to enjoy and that can be hard.

Recently, having taken Oliver skiing for a week, I wished I could take them both, but Harry wouldn't cope with that type of holiday, and Oliver deserves some time to enjoy his days without worrying about Harry's safety. The fact that I couldn't take them both and that I can't give them equal opportunities to enjoy the world makes me sad.

From the first moment I looked at Harry, I thought, *He's my boy and it's up to me to make sure he's safe.* He was, and still is so precious, and I think our bond has definitely grown stronger over the years. The baby years were hard with life in general and his operations. Part of me regrets the first balloon operation he had. Charlene holding him down while I injected his head as he screamed. All for nothing. I found that so hard.

Putting your child's life into someone else's hands is possibly the scariest thing a parent has to deal with, and it never gets easier. I know we have more decisions to make in the future, and weighing up the costs and benefits is something that I always find difficult. Making a decision for your own life is daunting enough, but the enormity of making decisions for someone else feels overwhelming at times.

What's been the hardest part of your journey?

Of all the disorders and conditions that Harry has, him being non-verbal is probably the hardest and most frustrating aspect of life that we have had to deal with. Not being able to comfort him, or understand his needs. Not knowing how his day was at school or what he'd really like to do at the weekend. It's always a guessing game, and I would love for him to be able to tell us how he's feeling so that we'd know for sure we are doing the right thing for him. It's definitely got easier as he's got older and communicates with us better, but I always think how much parents take for granted as they watch their children develop.

What advice would you give to other dads at the start of their own Altered Life journey?

My advice to other dads would be to talk to your partner, no matter what discomfort or arguments it might cause in the short term. Sometimes the words that are left unsaid have more destructive power than anything you could ever say to each other.

Listen to the advice that others give you but don't feel like you have to follow it all. Use your own judgement and be true to yourself and what you and your family need. Don't ever be scared or embarrassed to ask any questions. Write them down as you think of them or you will forget them, and don't feel intimidated by the professionals you meet. It's your child's life, and although they may be experts in their field, you are the expert on your child. It's your life too.

What are your thoughts on the future?

Right now, life is great and the boys are settled in both their homes. I know that we will have a lot more hurdles in front of us in the years to come, but Charlene and I are still a great team so I know it will be fine. I always will be there for Harry and Oliver. I'm their dad and they are my world.

When I look back, I try to focus on the positive aspects of our journey where I can, but even the tough times were worth it when I look at how happy and bubbly my boys are now. Both boys are amazing and always exceed their own and our expectations. Oliver is rapidly turning into a wonderful young man, and though Harry will always be a boy, I am incredibly proud of both of them.

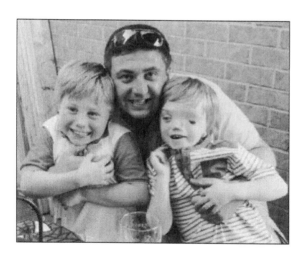

Acknowledgements

I would like to thank the following people for their support as I have lived and written my journey.

To my mum. Thank you for your unconditional love, even when I was hard to love. I honestly don't know what I would have done without you at my side. Thank you for always believing in me and never letting me give up on myself.

To Mark. Our boys amaze me every single day. I never expected our lives to change the way they did, but we created two unique, incredible people and I will always be grateful to you for them, and for our friendship that remains strong to this day.

To Andrew. For your unwavering love and support as I have spent so much time, energy and money writing and sharing my journey. Thank you for loving me and my boys and for giving me my happy ending.

To my nan for always believing that Harry was a gift sent to us for a very special reason and for being the best sidekick a girl could ever wish for. I miss you dearly and strive every single day to make you proud.

To my friends – the ones who have travelled the journey with me from the start and the incredible ones I have met along the way. Our lives are richer for having you in them.

For Emily and Colette who were my guinea pigs in reading and critiquing my book. Who better than the grammar police and the queen of articulation? Plus Grace and Sarah who were so patient with my endless "Does this sound right?' questions. Thank you all for your time and your honest feedback.

Thank you to my wonderful editor Alison Jack who refined my words but maintained my voice. Thanks also to Julia Gibbs for her fantastic proof reading and the team at Spiffing Covers for creating the cover of my book.

A huge thank you to Simon & Schuster Inc. and Jodi Picoult for permission to quote the passage from Handle with Care and to Emily Perl Kingsley for her permission to use 'Welcome to Holland'. My story wouldn't have been complete without sharing how profoundly your words helped me. I live in hope that maybe one day some of my own words will help another mother in the same way.

Finally the most important thank you of all – to my boys.

To Oliver – where do I begin? Thank you for understanding, for never complaining, for waiting in the wings at times when you deserved centre stage. You are the star of our show, my boy. Thank you for becoming such a caring, compassionate, loving and wonderful young man. I have no words for how proud and grateful I feel every day that you are my son – the greatest thing I ever did.

For Harry. Thank you for choosing me to be your mum. For teaching me so much about strength, life and myself. For showing me the true meaning of unconditional love. Our life together is seldom easy, but you make every day wonderful. Thank you for our altered life. You are my sunshine.

Printed in Great Britain
by Amazon

42201760R00184